STOMACH AND BOWEL DISORDERS

Stomach and Bowel Disorders

JAN DE VRIES

Foreword by **HAYLEY MILLS**

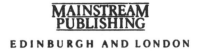
MAINSTREAM
PUBLISHING

EDINBURGH AND LONDON

First published in Great Britain in 1993 by
MAINSTREAM PUBLISHING COMPANY (EDINBURGH) LTD
7 Albany Street
Edinburgh EH1 3UG

Reprinted 1997, 1998, 1999

ISBN 1 85158 535 4 (cased)
ISBN 1 85158 534 6 (paperback)

A catalogue record for this book in available from the British Library

Typeset in Palatino by WEPS Electronic Publishing Systems, Scotland
Printed and bound in Finland by WSOY

Contents

Foreword

As Patron of the Jan de Vries Benevolent Trust, let me first say what an honour it is to be invited to write the foreword to this book.

The work of the Trust is centred around holistic forms of medicine, the best known being homoeopathy, osteopathy and acupuncture, which are increasingly being used in conjunction with orthodox medicine by the medical profession. This complementary medicine, as it is known, is successfully treating twentieth-century diseases such as Candida albicans, irritable bowel syndrome and ME by treating the person as a whole, as opposed to selective treatment. In the following pages Jan de Vries discusses reasons behind today's widespread health problems related to drinking, smoking, over-eating and, of course, stress, and the exciting medical options now available to us.

Jan de Vries is one of Europe's foremost practitioners of complementary medicine, and for over thirty years has helped bring holistic healthcare to a point where demand is greater than qualified practitioners can supply.

The Trust, set up in his name, aims to maintain and improve research and training into holistic medicine, and increase the

7

number of qualified practitioners who in turn are helping to build bridges between orthodox and complementary health-care. It also strives to provide patients with much needed financial support for both orthodox and complementary treatment.

This practical handbook will provide help and guidance to those people interested in complete health, and royalties from sales of this book go to the Trust.

HAYLEY MILLS
The Jan de Vries Benevolent Trust
18 Bristo Place
Edinburgh
EH1 1HA

Chapter 1

Abdominal Pain

There is no better place than at the beginning of the first chapter to relate a personal experience from 1987 which is relevant to the subject of his book. It had been quite a stressful year and I had had to make some extremely difficult decisions relating to patients as well as to my business. I was not sleeping very well at that time and I became somewhat alarmed by spells of inexplicable abdominal pain.

I often point out to patients that abdominal pain should never be ignored, because frequently this is a signal that something, somewhere, is not as it should be. I probably ignored the initial warnings because I was so busy, but I eventually reached the point where the pain became so obvious and persistent that I was forced to seek the help of a specialist. I had discussed the matter with a colleague with whom I had worked for many years and she insisted that I speak with a friend of hers. We spent the best part of a Sunday together and he made plenty of notes and thoroughly checked me over. Afterwards my colleague received the following report:

> You will recall our conversation regarding Jan de Vries. For the last couple of weeks he has had epigastric pain radiating into the lower part of his chest and on one occasion down his left arm. He finds that the discomfort comes on daily about 4 o'clock. His appetite is normal. There is no change in his weight.
>
> In the past he has been fairly well, apart from some left flank discomfort thought to be due to spastic bowel, and he has previously had an IVP for a suspected renal cal-

9

culus. Physical examination revealed a rather fit-looking man. Blood pressure was 145/185. The chest was normal to examination, apart from a slight end expiratory wheeze. He had no palpable lymph nodes. The heart was normal. He had epigastric tenderness on palpation. The central nervous system was intact.

The following investigations were carried out. An ECG was normal. Hb. 14.8 g/dl, W.C.C. 6.9, EST 1mm. Sodium and potassium were normal. His urea was slightly elevated at 9.4 mmol/l. but with a normal creatinine. I do not think that this result is of any major significance. Blood sugar, random, was normal. Urate normal. His liver enzymes were normal, Alk. Phos. normal. Serum proteins, calcium and cholesterol were all within the normal range.

A chest X-ray was done and looks normal, although I have not had the report. A gastroscopy was done and this showed a normal oesophagus. The stomach was essentially normal, apart from the pre-pyloric area where there was intense pre-pyloric oedema with haemorrhage. The endoscope was passed into the duodenum with some difficulty because of the spasm. In the duodenum there was widepsread haemorrhagic duodenitis with a small superficial ulcer in the duodenal cap. There is little doubt that Jan de Vries has had duodenal ulcer disease, probably for some time.

I have spoken with him as to advised treatment, but have not arranged to see him again. Obviously if problems continue I will be happy to do so.

Well, this report more or less reflects what can happen if we pay insufficient attention to our health. It was a feeble excuse to claim that I had been too busy looking after the well-being of so many other people. Deep down I had known that something was wrong, and my suspicions were confirmed by the tests. Stress was the cause of the abdominal pain, which eventually revealed itself as an ulcer.

Fortunately, there was no need for me to follow the advised drug treatment, because I knew perfectly well which natural remedies to select for my problems. This left me with the dilemma of finding the necessary recovery time, because many of my patients come from far afield and appointments are made a long time in advance. However, with some careful rescheduling, I managed to ease my workload slightly and I was rewarded; once I had been made to see reason, I worked very hard towards recovery.

The primary reason for including the report at the very beginning of this book is to stress the importance of paying attention to the alarm signals produced by the body. I stress this point in my book *Body Energy*, where I mention a number of examples of physical symptoms which indicate that some function or other is impaired. It is likely that a persistent niggling pain or a recurring bout of indigestion can alert us that something is wrong. It is easy to forget that today's stress can result in fairly serious future problems such as irritable bowel syndrome, an ulcer, or many other non-specific digestive problems. Too often it is an indication that we pay insufficient attention to sensible dietary management.

In my book *Nature's Gift of Food* I repeatedly remind the reader of the importance of food combining. It is vital that we learn to respect food, and allow ourselves the time to prepare our meals properly. Bear in mind that good nutrition is the foundation for good health, and that it, combined with stress management, are the 'pillars of health'. Of equal importance is good digestion and good absorption. When food enters the mouth, it passes through the stomach and enters the duodenum, and this is where my personal problems originated.

In my case the duodenum could not cope with the stress or with the little time I allowed myself for a meal break. Although I should be grateful that according to the report I was considered a reasonably fit man for my age, I still experienced considerable problems. I had to admit that I had paid insufficient attention to my own well-being. Better than most people, I should know that the most important aspects of food balancing are maintaining the balance of amino acids, glucose and essential fatty acids. This knowledge had not been reflected in my dietary programme.

Bearing in mind that some carcinogenic conditions may well have started with either abdominal pains or a duodenal or gastric ulcer, we must conclude that food absorption is of vital importance. Many of the thousands of patients I have seen over the years have been worried about indigestion; personally, I am much more concerned about absorption. If the absorption is deficient, a number of problems can arise. If absorption is correct, and food passes through the small intestine, the residual waste reaches the large intestine from where it can leave the body by an elimination process.

Remember, however, that the intake of inadequate food will result in impaired blood circulation. If a person is troubled with constipation, well-functioning blood circulation is of great importance. The circulation affects the functions of every organ, including the liver and the heart, and this will influence the cell renewal process. The constant reproduction of cells, good or bad, is an ongoing process, and to favourably influence this process is a constant battle to provide the body with healthy cells. This is where I was so lucky and why I managed to continue working long hours before I was fully recovered. I very consciously adapted my diet and lifestyle in the knowledge that adequate nutrition should contain plenty of amino acids, glucose, essential fatty acids, enzymes, vitamins, minerals and oxygen. No matter how busy one's life is, one should always set aside some time to exercise in the fresh air. This encourages the elimination of waste matter through the blood, so that the function of the kidneys, lungs and skin is not impaired. It can usually be seen at a glance whether a person has good health or not.

I never tire of pointing out the three major dangers to our health, which I refer to as 'the three S's', namely, stress, sugar and salt. A healthy constitution depends to a large extent on nutrition and relaxation, which allows the body to get on with the job for which it has been so excellently designed. I admit that in some of the tropical countries I have visited, I have sometimes found the slow pace of life of the natives slightly irritating. Few seemed to suffer stomach or bowel disorders, however, because their bodies were allowed sufficient time to enable the chemical process that is required for good digestion and absorption to take place.

In using the word 'chemical', it is essential to specify what kind of chemicals we are referring to. These should be 'responsible chemicals': in my work I have come to appreciate the importance of food that has life in it. The roughage in food will help the army of healthy cells to overcome the sick cells in our body in order that we get the best out of life. It must be understood that there is no place for food containing colourings and additives.

Thinking back to my statement on the 'pillars of health' that are necessary for a chemical balance, the aspects to consider are nutrition, digestion, elimination, circulation and relaxation. These are the factors that will determine our physical well-being and our mental and emotional state. Some of the problems discussed in this book can linger for long periods before they are checked, and abdominal pains can easily be an early signal of developing irritable bowel syndrome, which is often connected with the non-acceptance of an existing problem.

My first reaction to the report from the specialist who examined me for stomach disorders was 'Why me?'. This question is often asked when illness or disease occurs, and it indicates a general refusal to accept that something is wrong. There is a voice at the back of our mind which maintains that such things only happen to other people, not to us. We egotistically refuse to acknowledge the implications of our lifestyle. Certainly, in my own case, I deserved to pay a price for my obstinate refusal to give enough attention to my health. Upon consideration I could have come up with an instant answer to the question 'Why me?'. It really was my own fault and it only needed some common sense to correct the situation.

Illness and disease are very closely associated with self-awareness, possibly something in our lifestyle, which may be either imbalanced or too demanding. We eventually reach the crucial point where we either decide to do something positive about the problem, or else resign ourselves to the fact and adapt our lifestyle accordingly. So many times I hear patients remark that they may as well try to learn to live with their problem. They seem to forget that, given half a chance, this problem will take over their lives. Acceptance in this case does not provide us with a sensible answer. If we have a problem we must find a way of overcoming it, paying heed to the alarm signals sent out by the body. These are like calls for help in the only language the body knows.

We know that stress, nervousness and a negative mental attitude influence and cause imbalance in the immune system. This will reflect in the chemical industry of the body, as the mind and the consciousness are closely associated. There is little point in agreeing that stress affects the immune system and then ignoring the issue. It may need some courage to admit that the body does not function as it should and if we are prepared to view ourselves objectively, we can discover what must be done to change the situation so that we can enjoy a more worthwhile life. I once heard a lecturer make the apt comparison that 'an ill person is like a caterpillar, while a healthy person is like a butterfly'. This saying rather appealed to me.

To repeat what was established at the start of the chapter, we are now more likely to realise that abdominal pain may be a symptom of an existing disease. It could result from a multitude of disorders and indicate serious problems such as ulcers, appendicitis, obstructions, pancreatitis and other conditions which I will discuss later in this book.

I must use this opportunity to emphasise the importance of nutrition. First we must have an answer to the following questions:

- Is food a means of self-destruction?
- Is the purpose of food one of indulgence or enjoyment?
- Should food be regarded as an ally to help us to obtain and maintain good health?

Consider the facts:

- One third of the world's population suffers from food shortages and therefore lacks proper nutrition.
- A further third of the population suffers from adverse effects brought about by food indulgence and excess of food.

Ask yourself if there is enough 'real' food in what you eat. Do we judge our diet by the quality of food or by its quantity? Remember the old saying that a little quality goes a long way. Much of our food contains little or no goodness and is therefore only suitable as a 'filler'. Even if the food has quality in the first place, do our preparation methods destroy this goodness? Too often problems arise because we allow our food intake to adversely affect our cholesterol level or our body weight, and by doing so we create an ideal opportunity for the development of a Candida albicans condition (this is discussed in more detail in Chapter 15).

Healthy eating means regular mealtimes with food that has life in it. Only eat when hungry, and chew the food thoroughly. Many abdominal problems are self-inflicted because no attention is paid to these simple ground rules. You may know the expression 'we are what we eat', which contains a lot of truth. There have been many changes in nutritional ideas over the past few decades: it is quite baffling to learn that in the 1960s a distinguished Harley Street specialist started prescribing a diet rich in bran for patients with diverticulitis. Yet, at the same time, he confided in them that if this prescription became common knowledge he would be ridiculed by his colleagues. Now, fortunately, every medical authority recognises the importance of fibre in our diet. Despite the relatively recent changes in nutritional ideas and the publicity they receive, we still see abdominal conditions which have been allowed to get out of hand because of poor nutritional management. The alarm signals have been ignored.

With persistent abuse it does not take long for a stomach ulcer to develop, and it is sad to note that the statistics claim that approximately one in ten people suffer from this problem at some stage of their life, primarily because the early warning signs have been misinterpreted. At one time doctors used to advise ulcer patients to follow a milk or a bland diet to neutralise stomach acid, although there was very little evidence that such steps were effective. Nowadays ulcer sufferers are advised to take regular meals which are rich in fibre, while avoiding fried and highly spiced foods. Even with non-specific abdominal pains it very often helps to avoid alcohol, drinks containing caffeine, spices, salt and sometimes sugar, too.

Recently, it has been scientifically proved that food has a mechanism for adjusting living bodies to maintain health. The defensive or immune system needs more understanding, but we do know that various organs and their functions within the body support each other and interrelate. For example, the nervous system and the internal secretion system need to work in harmony in order for the body's defence system to be effective. The air around us contains a great number of bacteria and if these were to invade, the body would start a concerted fight against them. If the body is defeated in this battle, we may get a cold, which could result in pneumonia. If there is an inflammatory reaction or an allergy, we may experience abdominal discomfort. So to keep our health in optimum condition we have to protect the balance. Certain nutritional elements are necessary for this.

For some time now I have given a leaflet with nutritional advice to patients with stomach and abdominal disorders, containing both general and specific dietary guidelines. Information has been added and deleted over the years and the dietary advice is preceded by an introduction. The contents of this leaflet are given below.

Nutritional advice for stomach and abdominal disorders

Stomach and intestinal conditions can present themselves in many guises, for example, gastritis (inflammation of the stomach lining), stomach ulcers, duodenal ulcers, colitis, enteritis, and so on. For all these conditions, as well as for those not specifically mentioned, the golden rule is to ensure that the food that is eaten is in as natural a state as possible. The science of naturopathy is based on the assumption that natural food is essential.

It should be understood that particularly in the case of abdominal disorders, the cause, symptoms and effects of the various conditions vary greatly from one person to the next. Therefore, an individual approach is required in dietary management and any general statements should be considered as no more than guidelines. Everyone with abdominal complaints ought to adapt their food intake according to the diseased digestive organs, that is, according to their physical and psychic condition, and thus it is recommended that they seek the advice of a qualified dietician. In most cases additional medical care will be desired, if not essential, for example, to supplement intestinal bacteria, the use of biological or homoeopathic remedies, herbal therapy, respiratory or movement therapy, psychotherapy, and so on.

The following guidelines are therefore no more than a basic foundation which may be complemented in a manner which is specific to the condition of the person concerned.

The aim of the diet is primarily to obtain peace, peace for the stomach and intestines to allow these organs time to recover. In the second place the intention is to ensure an efficient supply of the essential nutrients such as vitamins, minerals, enzymes, and so on, required for recovery. These nutrients are richly present in raw foods, but are seriously diminished by cooking, frying or baking. Thirdly, the diet is responsible for the re-establishment of the bacterial balance in the intestines. Combined, these factors enable the healing process to function.

General advice
(1) Eat slowly and masticate the food thoroughly.
(2) It is essential to avoid alcohol, tobacco, tea, coffee, cocoa, chocolate and meat extracts. Smoking is strictly forbidden.
(3) For a period of two to three weeks all unnatural ingredients must be avoided.
(4) All products containing sugar or white flour are forbidden, and sometimes also honey. (Avoidance of sugar and white flour, in whichever shape or form, is one of the basic dietary guidelines for stomach disorders. Even those foods that contain only little sugar can cause detrimental, or at the least unpleasant, results, such as bloatedness and flatulence.)
    The following is an example of the foods to be avoided: white sugar, brown (cane and demerara) sugar, white bread, cakes, biscuits, all pasta products such as noodles, macaroni and spaghetti, desserts, custard, and so on. (It must be stressed that unless this advice is followed, in most cases no improvement in the condition should be anticipated.)
(5) Not only solids, but also vegetable or fruit juices, should be 'chewed' in order to combine the food with saliva, which aids the digestion.

Nutrition instructions
(1) Fruit and vegetables
    Raw fruit should be eaten as a starter or as a main course, but never after the meal. Initially, fruit should be liquidised, and even this should be

17

'chewed' to prepare it for assimilation by the digestive system.

At the start of the course, raw vegetables should be
consumed in liquidised form, for example, carrot,
tomato and vegetable juices. Later the vegetables
may be puréed, starting with carrot, tomato and
chicory, vegetables that are easily digestible, always remembering to 'chew' the vegetable purée.
Then one is allowed to progress to raw green leaf
vegetables.

A mixture of raw vegetables should be eaten as a
first course and may contain a choice of radishes,
spinach, white and red cabbage, endive, lettuce,
cauliflower, and so on. The first course should consist of at least one third of the meal. (If the patient
appears to be intolerant to mixing vegetables and
fruit in one meal, this should be taken into consideration when planning a menu.)

(2) Drinks

No tea, coffee or chocolate allowed, nor sweetened
soft drinks. Freshly squeezed fruit juices are recommended, which may be diluted with linseed decoc-
tion if digestive problems are experienced.

(3) Bread and grains

Wholemeal and coarse wheaten bread are recommended, as are crispbread and ryebread. However,
this should be very gradually introduced into the
diet if it was not part of the patient's original diet.
It goes without saying that these breads should be
chewed very thoroughly, producing plenty of
saliva.

Dr Vogel's Muesli – a combination of grains, nuts
and dried fruits – may be used to substitute bread
at certain meals. Refined grain products such as
white bread, cake, semolina, macaroni, spaghetti,
and so on, must be considered as de-naturalised
products and as such are partly responsible for the
many abdominal diseases experienced nowadays,
and therefore should always be avoided.

(4) Potatoes

Good potatoes – especially those organically grown
– deserve a rightful place in anyone's diet, as they
are a rich source of starch, mineral salts and vitamin

C. Peeled potatoes lose many of their nutrients in the cooking process, however, and it is therefore much wiser to steam or bake potatoes. It may be helpful to know that most of the nutrients are retained if the potatoes are peeled after having been boiled.

(5) Meat and fish

Meat is acid-inducing and as such burdens the digestive system unnecessarily. It also impedes the anti-fermentation process which is essential for natural healing. To a lesser extent, this is also the case with fish. It is therefore advised that patients with abdominal complaints avoid both meat and fish.

(6) Milk, butter and fat

It is widely known that roasted or fried foods are more difficult to digest. On the other hand, cold-pressed oils are more easily assimilated and often people with stomach disorders benefit from taking one or two spoonfuls of cold-pressed olive oil before breakfast in the morning.

Most milk fats and butter are well tolerated and in many cases buttermilk and yoghurt are more agreeable than full-fat unskimmed milk. Recently it has been recognised that fromage frais is particularly suitable for stomach disorders.

Diet Plan

It has already been pointed out that only dietary guidelines can be given for abdominal disorders, because a patient with a stomach ulcer will require a different dietary composition from a patient suffering from dyspepsia or over-acidity. The length of time a person has suffered the symptoms must also be taken into consideration.

In serious or acute cases a fast of three or four days (longer for an ulcer) is recommended, followed by one week of very easily digested foods, for example, porridge, grated apple, banana, wheatgerm, muesli and herbal tea. Gradually carrot juice, wholewheat bread and mashed potato may be introduced. When the person reacts well to this régime and is free of pain and discomfort, the time is right for a more varied menu, still taking account of the previous general instructions.

Complementary therapies

It must be realised that a consequent adoption of these guidelines sometimes may appear to cause further deterioration. This, however, can be explained as a natural reaction of the body – in other words a healing crisis. Therefore it is advisable to follow this régime under the guidance of a practitioner.

General lifestyle

(1) As the digestive system requires rest, it is therefore wise to rest during and after the meal, physically and mentally.

(2) Adhere wherever possible to regular mealtimes.

(3) Remember that a regular bowel movement is essential.

(4) Relax and avoid worry. Psychological balance is important.

(5) Walking and breathing exercises are beneficial.

(6) Do not smoke and ensure a good oxygen supply in the working environment and bedroom.

(7) Take care of a good circulation and warm feet. If desired use hydrotherapy.

Chapter 2

Dyspepsia and Indigestion

A young mother, the wife of a general practitioner, made an appointment at the clinic. When I first saw her I noticed that although she was very attractive, she looked really ill. She told me that her husband had done everything he could. A friend of his, a gastroenterologist, had also looked into her case, but it had all been to no avail. The final conclusion was that she suffered from dyspepsia, and although I agreed that this was the correct diagnosis, her condition had not improved. This affliction can best be described as a digestive disorder causing a pressing feeling in the abdominal area, often coupled with a diminished appetite and an unpleasant taste in the mouth. Her husband had asked me to examine his wife to find out if there was any chance that she might benefit from acupuncture treatment.

First of all I had a long chat with her and she was most co-operative. We discussed various aspects of her life: stress, sensitivities and emotional involvement with the children and her ageing parents, worries about her husband's busy lifestyle, and so on. I explained that sensitive people are more likely to experience dyspepsia: often early alarm bells are ignored because such a person is likely to be very involved in the life and care of others, taking their responsibilities very seriously.

With mutual trust and co-operation we managed to get this patient's problem under control and ever since that time her husband and I have been firm friends, despite the differences in our approach to medicine. This all took place quite some time ago, but to this day he will still occasionally refer some of his patients to me.

Let us first of all have a look at what takes place in the digestive process in the stomach. Digestion includes all the activities of the digestive tracts, involving the preparing of food to be absorbed by the body and the rejection of its residues. I often point out that whatever foods are imported, the remains should be exported preferably within a period of twenty-four hours. If this does not happen we may well experience problems. Another, slightly more direct, saying is: 'what begins at the lips ends at the rectum'. The preliminary chemical breakdown of food takes place in the mouth, before it passes to the stomach. The digestive tract has to cope with many different foodstuffs and is therefore often grossly overworked. We expect too much of it and sometimes don't chew our food properly, thus placing even more of a burden on the digestion. Our choice of food too often lacks the proper composition, hence the importance of sensible food combining. It does not make sense to overload the digestive tract, as this will cause contractions of the circular muscles.

When food has arrived at the lower end of the oesophagus, it passes through a valve – the cardiac sphincter – which controls entry to the stomach. The sphincter is an opening with a circular set of muscles. When there is too much contraction, possibly resulting from excess stress or tension, the sphincter may not function correctly and therefore will not allow free entry of the food into the passageway. Indigestive discomfort is the result, manifesting itself as burping, flatulence or eructations. These are not only uncomfortable experiences, but are also considered unsociable. Stomach gas, derived from air swallowed with food or drink, builds up in the upper part of the stomach until the cardiac sphincter allows it to escape into the oesophagus.

The important function of the stomach is to act as a store for ingested food, and the stomach – which consists of a J-shaped bag – can be divided into three parts: the cardiac area, the fundic area and the pyloric area. These three areas are completely distinct from one another, and the whole stomach has a muscular wall enabling it to produce a churning action which breaks up food and ensures a beneficial chemical breakdown. The muscular contraction depends on the nervous system, in particular the vagus nerve. It also controls the production and secretion of digestive juices. Its effectiveness is subject to the correct acid and alkaline balance. Hydrochloric acid (HCl), an important factor in the digestion of food, is present and the stomach can produce a large amount of this strong acid.

In my book *Nature's Gift of Food* I stress the fact that the acid-alkaline system deserves our attention. Too much or too little acid can cause problems, and a balance should be maintained. What the reader should understand is that if we keep our food as natural as possible, we have a better chance of maintaining this balance. One of the best foods for balancing the acid-alkaline system is rice. Another natural substance that acts as an excellent balancer, especially if there is too much wind in the stomach, is the cornflower – *Centaurium umbellatum*. This was certainly a great help for the doctor's wife I mentioned at the start of this chapter. Centaurium is one of the most helpful herbs for stomach or indigestion problems. Dr Vogel recommends Centaurium for the treatment of digestive irregularities, lack of appetite, a weak and/or sour stomach, and for inflammation of the mucous membranes of the stomach.

Another very helpful remedy is Betaine Hydrochloride with pepsin which helps maintain the correct pH balance in the stomach – particularly useful for the over-60s – and provides pepsin, the stomach's protein-splitting enzyme. An imbalance in the hydrochloric acid level can result in dyspepsia and ulcers, often induced by poor eating habits. Too much acidity can erode parts of the stomach wall, causing ulcers, and in the worst case haemorrhage may necessitate surgery. Pepsin starts the breakdown of the long chain molecules of the proteins and, as a result, this Nature's Best remedy is often helpful.

We should now turn our attention to the stomach cells which are protected by a coating of mucus secreted by the mucous cells. This coating forms a barrier between the gastric juices and the cells. The gastric secretion needs the enzyme renin, possibly better known as a milk-curdling agent. Its function is to break up the molecular chains of the protein casein, which is found in milk. This product is unfortunately often lacking in the average diet, and therefore I often advise drinking Molkosan with a meal, and especially with the main meal of the day.

Molkosan is a Bioforce remedy produced from fresh Alpine whey by a natural fermentation process. It contains in concentrated form all the important minerals found in fresh whey such as magnesium, potassium and calcium. Molkosan is rich in natural dextrorotatory L(=)-lactic acid, which, in health-oriented nutrition as well as natural healing methods, has a special significance. It is beneficial in protecting against skin diseases, oral infections and tonsilitis. It also increases the effects of rutin.

Molkosan should be used as a substitute for vinegar in salad dressings or by adding one tablespoon to a glass of mineral water for a refreshing cold drink. It can also be added to vegetable juices for a little extra zip. Dr Vogel recommends it for the following purposes:

Internally
- weight control, as it improves metabolism
- encouragement and maintenance of a healthy intestinal flora
- indigestion
- stimulation of the secretion of gastric acid
- sore throat – gargle with 1 part Molkosan and 2 parts water for soothing relief and faster recovery
- mouth disinfectant – using the same dilution as for gargling

Externally – as a disinfectant for:
- minor cuts and abrasions
- athlete's foot and other skin and nail mycosis (diluted 1 to 1 with water)
- eczema and skin impurities (use externally and internally)

So, apart from the enzymes renin and casein we look at the third stomach enzyme, which is gastric lipase. This acts on the butterfat molecules of milk, splitting them into smaller parts, and adults especially rely on the enzyme found in the small intestine to perform this function. The gastric secretions are under the control of the nervous and hormonal systems. The hormone gastrine is secreted by the pyloric region of the stomach when protein foods are present and by the stimulation of nerves. For any problem in this process Nature's Best remedy Pancreatin is highly recommended. It is composed of cold-pressed viobin which contains three pancreatic enzymes: lipase, protease and amylase. I often prescribe this remedy in conjunction with Dr Vogel's Gastronol, a multi-ingredient antacid homoeopathic medicine for the treatment of intestinal problems, especially diarrhoea, stomach cramps, flatulence and acid indigestion.

When food is thoroughly mixed, the peristaltic waves at about the middle of the stomach begin to push the partly digested food towards the pyloric sphincter. This is another valve formed by a muscular ring which prevents food passing into the duodenum, whilst the first part goes to the small intestine. Pressure in the stomach is increased mainly by the peristaltic waves and it takes about two to six hours for the stomach to empty all its contents. One should know that food rich in carbohydrates leaves in a few hours, followed by protein-rich food, while the fatty food is the last to leave.

The stomach in itself does very little in the process of absorbing nutrients from food into the bloodstream. Water and some salts pass through the stomach wall, but the major breakdown and absorption process takes place in the small intestines, subject to a healthy digestive system.

Indigestion may only be a matter of burping, gas-formation or flatulence. Dyspepsia, which is mostly a follow-up, includes nausea, heartburn, upper abdominal pain, a sense of fullness and a feeling of abdominal distension. While indigestion may be triggered by eating too much, most symptoms result from an ultra-gastric motor activity. Sometimes nervousness or anxiety, fear or shock, constipation, smoking or alcohol abuse may lead to a severe dyspepsia problem. Not only flatulence, but also nausea or heartburn may result, which can lead to retention or regurgitation of food and a gastric acidity which comes up in the throat. Flatulence is the accumulation of wind and gas, and this is often experienced when there is unusual nervousness or fermentation in the bowels, when food is not properly digested or absorbed. The abdominal cramps or pain which are the first indication are often ignored in the early stages. The nauseous feeling of a dyspeptic patient may be significant, especially if it is linked with vomiting. Action is essential and in such cases the homoeopathic remedy nux vomica is of great help. These problems should be correctly diagnosed, as the distension of the

25

stomach may also indicate an allergy or an active Candida albicans problem (see Chapter 15).

Dyspepsic indigestion has a host of names and as many causes. Apart from the food-related factors, there are others which should not be overlooked. Much information was gained from studying accident victims who had suffered severe injuries and who were left with a permanent opening in the abdomen that exposed the stomach lining. It was observed that the stomach lining responded exactly the same way as a face does in an emotional state. When the face blushed, the stomach blushed as well. This confirms the experiences of the doctor's wife who felt that her condition was subject to emotional circumstances and influences. Digestive or dyspepsia problems can also result from illness, and after a period of being unwell it may be wise to take a digestive aid such as Pancreatin or Centaurium, with daily use of Molkosan to correctly balance the digestive system.

At recent meetings and lectures I have paid special attention to culinary herbs such as rosemary, fennel, aniseed and sage. Chamomile or peppermint teas are also helpful. If nausea is frequently experienced, it should be remembered that some freshly grated ginger root gives relief.

In the days when I travelled regularly with Dr Vogel we studied the habits of people in various parts of the world who were unfamiliar with such problems. I remember a particular journey when we discovered a herb that was used as a means of prevention and as a result of that discovery Arabiaforce was developed. Arabiaforce is an excellent remedy which I prescribe almost daily, not only as a preventative but also as an answer to many digestive or dyspepsia problems. This herbal remedy has been developed for the general purpose of stimulating stomach activity and for the promotion of the appetite. In particular it is prescribed for dyspepsia, sub-acidic gastritis, stomach cramps, nausea and as a stimulant of biliary flow. Arabiaforce contains the following herbs:

Aloe capensis	Aloe
Nux cola	Cola nut
Cortex chinae succ.	Peruvian bark
Fructus auranti immat.	Bitter orange

Rhizoma calami	Sweet myrtle
Gentiana lutea	Yellow gentian
Gummi myrrhae	Myrrh
Olibanum elect.	Frankincense

With the help of the remedies mentioned much pain and discomfort can be forestalled, especially if timely attention is paid to the early distress signals.

Chapter 3

Hiatus Hernia

On one and the same day I had the opportunity to witness the evidence of the widely different approaches of orthodox and alternative medicine. Yet, at the same time, I also saw why the two sciences should complement each other rather than be considered in opposition. My first patient in the consulting room that day was someone I have known for many years. In his stressful life as a journalist, and later as an editor, he developed problems which resulted in hiatus hernia. This medical condition is a defect where the sphincter between the oesophagus and the stomach is displaced from its normal site at the point level with the diaphragm where the oesophagus joins the stomach.

There are two types of hiatus hernia: the sliding type and the para-oesophageal type. The sliding type of hernia slips up into the chest and can cause very considerable discomfort, with burping and food repeating itself. This type of hernia is not a major medicinal problem and can often be treated by a healthy dietary approach, by eating small meals very slowly and masticating the food thoroughly. Often this problem is a side-effect of obesity. One's posture during mealtimes is also important. A sliding hernia rarely needs surgery, but is unfortunately rather common.

The para-oesophageal hiatus hernia, on the other hand, is medically much more serious. Although sometimes no larger than a minor hairline crack, severe discomfort and considerable damage can be the result. Quite often in such cases, surgery will have to be performed, but it is not an easy operation since a disproportionately large part of the body requires to be opened up.

It was this latter type of hernia that had been diagnosed in my patient: he sported an enormous scar which was the result of a hiatus hernia operation. Unfortunately, at the time he had never questioned the doctor's verdict that a surgical operation was essential and, without seeking a second opinion, he had followed the surgeon's advice. I am not proclaiming that surgery is never required, but I firmly believe that in quite a few cases hiatus hernia can be overcome with less dramatic measures. This belief was confirmed that same day, when I saw a gentleman with a very similar problem. It was eventually proved that this gentleman needed only a single osteopathic treatment session to overcome his problem.

As so often before, I had reason to be grateful to my teachers who had trained me so effectively. One of them was Gonstead from the USA, a well-informed and inspired teacher and first-class manipulative therapist. For both kinds of hiatus hernia, it was he who taught me to manipulate the affected area, from which so many patients have benefited over the years. I couldn't guess at how many patients I have been able to help, but I can assure you that the treatment is totally painless and most effective. Very seldom do I have to refer a hiatus hernia patient for surgery, as I am nearly always able to help with this simple manipulative treatment. Over the years I have been able to teach many medical students and doctors how this particular manipulative adjustment should be performed, so that in turn they will be able to help their patients to overcome this problem.

This fact does not mean that the hiatus hernia patient, who is very possibly the victim of some of the effects described in the two earlier chapters, does not need to pay extra attention to his or her diet. Understandably, the first recommendation for obese people is to lose weight. Those who have the constant urge to burp and who experience the uncomfortable sensation of food being obstructed, need to consider some form of digestive aid such as Centaurium. Also useful in such cases is the remedy Gentiana. This is another product of the Bioforce range, and contains *Gentiana lutea* (yellow gentian). It is specifically recommended for digestive problems and for liver and gall bladder dysfunctions.

Sometimes healing can be accelerated and enhanced by taking a calcium supplement. Dr Vogel's calcium preparation Urticalcin is one of the very best. This is a homoeopathic calcium and silicic acid supplement for use when a lack of calcium is indicated. Apart from building and strengthening the bones, it aids brittle nails and hair loss. It is often recommended during pregnancy and while nursing, and it has a preventative effect on the build-up of excessive amounts of acid in the body. The composition of Urticalcin is as follows:

Urtica dioica
Silicea
Calcarea carbonica
Calcarea phosphorica
Natrum phosphorica

Many years ago I remember Dr Vogel telling me that every doctor faces the same problem of how to obtain the maximum absorption of calcium into the blood supply. At some time he noticed a bunch of stinging nettles and realised that if he were to fall into the patch of nettles he would receive the best calcium injections possible. With that realisation he created the remedy Urticalcin, which has been a blessing for many people.

Another plant that has great medicinal properties is the hemp nettle or *Galeopsis ochroleuca*. This plant is the main ingredient in a remedy of the same name and this herbal preparation is ideally suited for the treatment of minor fractures. Galeopsis and Urticalcin are a wonderful combination for problems such as hiatus hernia.

Sometimes, when I am in a restaurant and I look around me, I am not surprised at having such a large number of hiatus hernia patients. Food gets very little respect nowadays and when I see how much food is wasted, my heart still cries out when I think back to the dark days of Holland in the Second World War. In those days I was sometimes reduced to eating grass to still the hunger pains in my stomach. Yet, despite the great famine during those years, hiatus hernia was not a common medical condition that many doctors were asked about. The very little food that was available was savoured when any of it came our way. Nowadays we think nothing of over-eating or eating until we are completely sated. By eating excessively we encourage problems such as hiatus hernia through not properly digesting food. I have already pointed out that saliva is an excellent digestive agent; many cases of hiatus hernia are self-inflicted because of hastily eaten food. By insufficient chewing the digestive system is overworked and is unable to function correctly.

Most food intolerances can be overcome by healthy food combining, and food allergies may be detected by a process of dietary elimination. With a sensible attitude and a good balance, many digestive and abdominal complaints can be avoided.

Chapter 4

Gastritis

There are two kinds of gastritis, which are acute and chronic inflammations of the stomach. Acute gastritis is an inflammation of the mucosa of the stomach, the symptoms of which can be very sudden and violent. Acute gastritis can again be subdivided into four types. Firstly, there is acute simple gastritis, or exogenous gastritis. This can be brought about by smoking, drinking, the smell and fumes of creosote and tar products, soapy products, bromide, quinine, very hot foods, bacteria and any other toxic matter. Secondly, there are acute gastric infections which can be caused by flu, scarlet fever, pneumonia and other kinds of fever. Thirdly, acute corrosive gastritis is brought on by swallowing strong acids, potassium or salts, as in mercury, zinc or lead. Fourth is acute suppurative gastritis which can be caused by stomach infections, with the involvement of streptococcus, colon bacillus, and so on.

To deal effectively with acute gastritis several factors play a role. Very often, exogenous gastritis will respond rapidly to the juice of a raw potato. Here I make the assumption that the reader is aware of the fact that gastritis, duodenal gastric ulcers, eczema and psoriasis are all nurtured by a hyper-acidity of the stomach. When this condition has become so bad that the acid rises into the mouth, drinking the juice of a raw potato can be extremely effective. Grate a well-washed and scrubbed potato, without removing the skin, and extract the juice by pressing the grated potato through a sieve. There will not be much juice but it is an excellent remedy to deal with these problems. It is best taken first thing in the morning and should always be freshly prepared. If this juice is not totally effective, try some charcoal, preferably obtained from the lime tree, which is also a most effective supplement.

I would never hesitate to recommend Dr Vogel's remedy Centaurium. With gastric acidity we should realise that the possible consequences of jaundice and other liver problems are very real, and that these could eventually result in even more serious complaints. If I think that the patient will benefit, I often recommend Active Charcoal Tablets available from Nature's Best, which are a long-established supplement of specially prepared charcoal, also known for its medicinal property of absorbing intestinal gases.

In my book *Traditional Home and Herbal Remedies* I mention the health benefits of garlic. This herb is mostly used for culinary purposes, but for thousands of years it has been recognised as a potent natural remedy. It has one drawback, which cannot be immediately discounted, and that is its smell. Many suppliers of garlic pearls or tablets have tried to solve this problem by deodorising, and the latest solution is to leave the garlic exposed to the air so that it ages and loses some of its pungent odour. Nature's Best have the technology to do this, but the result would have been a supplement that did not deliver the benefits of natural garlic. This is because the deodorising process strips garlic of allicin, its main active ingredient. Now Nature's Best have developed the technology to minimise the odour without affecting its activity. Their garlic supplement Pure-Gar is very much closer to the nutritional profile of natural raw garlic than other supplements. The same manufacturer also supplies a garlic remedy which combines parsley, a herb which is a known antidote for the smell of garlic and an ideal supplement for those who find the use of garlic or garlic-based remedies socially unpleasant. For all forms of acute gastritis garlic is of tremendous help and I usually guide my patients in this direction.

For acute infections it is also advisable to take Dr Vogel's natural antibiotic Echinaforce. I wouldn't know what to do without this remedy, and numerous people will support me in this. Not so long ago, on a transatlantic flight, I sat next to a gentleman in whom I perceived all the signs of acute gastritis. The only thing I had in my hand-luggage was a bottle of

Echinaforce, because I never travel without this remedy. I persuaded this passenger to take some and before we landed he told me that already he felt slightly better. I would recommend any reader to make sure they have a bottle in the medicine cupboard at home and also to ensure that it is packed when travelling.

The other day I saw a patient who told me that very suddenly he had felt unwell, nauseous, with a coated tongue and a headache, and it was easy to diagnose acute gastritis. Acute *corrosive* gastritis is often more difficult to treat, because there may be a collapse or a tachycardia and the abdomen becomes very tender and rigid. Acute *infectious toxic* gastritis often occurs as a side-effect of food poisoning, and quick action is necessary. With acute *suppurative* gastritis we see a dry tongue, rapid pulse, fast breathing and vomiting. All such cases of gastritis benefit from Echinaforce in combination with Centaurium.

At this point I want to draw the reader's attention to Gastronol, a homoeopathic remedy in the Bioforce range, which was specifically designed by Dr Vogel for the treatment of stomach and intestinal upsets such as diarrhoea, stomach cramps, flatulence and acid indigestion. For acute gastritis attacks these remedies are very valuable.

A serious suppurative gastritis case is more difficult to deal with, and sometimes surgery may be required. At all times the advice of doctors or practitioners should be followed, as quite often bed rest is necessary. Do not forget, however, that diet is always an important factor. With corrosive gastritis the treatment must be very quick, and immediate neutralisation of the offensive action is necessary. In most cases immediate bed rest is prescribed and in the case of gastric perforation, emergency surgical repair is needed.

Chronic gastritis is quite a different complaint. This is often caused by a chronic inflammation of the gastric mucosa. Here again there are three types, namely atrophic, superficial and hypertropic. Patients with chronic gastritis often suffer from a complete lack of stomach hydrochloric acid, a condition known as achlorhydria. This most common chronic gastritis occurs where the parietal cells have been destroyed by the atrophy of the gastric mucosa. Often cancer of the stomach is characterised by achlorhydria, mainly because the tumour envelops the cells so that they no longer function. This problem also occurs with pernicious anaemia, when no hydrochloric acid is produced, although the condition may respond favourably to vitamin B_{12} injections.

In chronic gastritis there is often an ulceration, and mucosal haemorrhages may be frequent. Patients often complain about sensations ranging from fullness to nausea, vomiting or loss of weight, and all the problems associated with ulcers.

Diagnosis of gastritis is mostly done by exclusion. In cases of a high gastric acidity with ulcer-like symptoms, it usually suggests a hypertropic gastritis, where symptomatically gastric acidity is higher than normal.

A qualified practitioner or doctor will be able to advise on the correct treatment for the diagnosed form of gastritis. Diet is always important for an abdominal or intestinal upset and highly spiced food should always be avoided. Drinking, smoking and drugs may have adverse effects, too. It should also be remembered that supplementary vitamins are of benefit and for these conditions I frequently suggest that the patient takes one or two tablets daily of Health Insurance Plus from Nature's Best. Besides vitamins, minerals and trace elements are also required, and for this purpose, preparations that contain zinc, iron and/or selenium are most favoured. Rarely is sufficient zinc obtained from our food intake and according to leading nutrition researchers, such as Dr Carl Pfeiffer MD PhD, more people find it difficult to obtain enough zinc than any other mineral.

Soils deficient in zinc have reduced the levels available in plant foods, and any zinc which remains could be removed by food processing. High levels of calcium and phyates, found in plant foods, are thought to block absorption of zinc from food. The body's store of zinc may be threatened by missing meals or fasting. The most reliable sources of zinc are shellfish, herring and meat, and quite rightly many vegetarians and people on a wholefood diet take zinc supplements. Smokers, alcohol-drinkers, users of the contraceptive pill, elderly people and athletes (as the mineral is lost in perspiration) are also well advised to take extra zinc.

Zinc is best known for its role in growth and tissue repair and also in the immune system, so it is vital that children and adolescents receive enough of this mineral. Zinc is not only required for overall growth, but is particularly important for the healthy function of reproductive organs and the prostate gland, as it is a component of semen.

These functions only scratch the surface of the importance of zinc, however, since this mineral is involved in hundreds of metabolic pathways. Some of these maintain vision and our senses of smell and taste. Others deal with the digestion of carbohydrates and the balance of blood-sugar controlling insulin, the absorption of other nutrients, such as vitamins A and the B-complex vitamins, and cell metabolism.

Zinc achieves so much by becoming a part of many different chemical catalysts or enzymes. It is one of our most important antioxidants, as part of the major antioxidant enzyme superoxide dismutase, and it protects cells from the damage caused by oxidising fats.

I have already mentioned the possible effects of a lack of hydrochloric acid. This may be supplemented, except of course in the case of hypertropic gastritis, which needs a different approach. As always, I am compelled to point out the importance of a healthy diet, especially the use of fresh fruit and vegetables. In order to combat and prevent the development of nitrozymes, which are cancer-producing agents, we know that it is essential to de-activate the nitrates and amines. This can be most effectively achieved by the vitamins C and E, and sometimes it is preferential to take these separately in a dosage prescribed by the practitioner. Chronic gastritis, especially if achlorhydria is diagnosed, is greatly helped by supplementary vitamin C and vitamin E, as well as by hydrochloric tablets.

Often gastritis problems can lead to more serious complaints and it is sad to discover that the initial discomfort has resulted from an unbalanced diet or from stress. We used to think that people with stressful positions were more prone to gastritis attacks, but this does not seem to be the case any longer. In the 1930s research was carried out where monkeys were trained to give other monkeys electric shocks, which resulted in ulcers. Later, the Rand Corporation studied the incidence of gastric problems in air traffic controllers and other people who worked in stressful occupations, and found them no more prone to ulcers and gastric problems than the general population. In the early 1900s the ratio of ulcer incidents among the general public was 4:1 in males. According to the Director for the Centre of Ulcer Research and Education at the Veterans' Administration Hospital in Los Angeles, this has since decreased. It is not known why the number of women with ulcers is steadily increasing, though a possible reason could be smoking.

All gastric problems, including ulcers (which have the highest incidence in the protective lining of the stomach) may be due to an imbalance in acid-controlling substances, and related to an acid-alkaline diet. Some acids are necessary for digestion, because acid converts pepsinogen to pepsin, an enzyme that degrades proteins into amino acids and eventually into glycogen, which is stored in the liver to maintain the blood-sugar level. Then it is secreted in response to the acetylcholine from the vagus nerve gastrin, from the anterim of the stomach, or histadine. Each of these substances have receptors or cells in the stomach lining. When the two join together acid is released, providing the individual's ability to secrete hydrochloric acid is active.

I once attended a conference in the USA where my friend Betty Lee Morales stated in her lecture that scientists are not sure why, but when something goes wrong, there is too much acid and it begins to eat into the stomach or duodenum, where partially digested foods are deposited. By 1977, when antacids were one of the largest-selling products in the world, the scientist Dajani said: 'We thought that acid was the culprit, so we developed drugs to inhibit the body's ability to secrete it; but now we recognise that we need some acid to help sterilise bacteria, amongst many other things.' A gradual decline in the body's production of hydrochloric acid is normal. At the age of forty most people require a digestive aid. If antacids give relief, they can also cause problems, as is now recognised. Old-time practitioners prescribed cider vinegar, thus ensuring acidity. By way of urine tests alkalinity can be monitored, and it is now recognised that the alkaline and acid balance can easily be upset. One of my patients had taken cider vinegar for a long time and eventually she was diagnosed as having a perforation of the stomach lining. So careful advice from qualified doctors or practitioners is very necessary.

Bearing in mind some of the body functions and considering the minerals that are an essential part of the human body, there is still much to learn about the acid condition of the body. In the past chemists have listed thirty-six acids that are contained in the human body and have expressed various opinions on these acids. For a better understanding a brief explanation of the nature of minerals and acids in the human body is required.

First, let us consider the three essential gases – oxygen, nitrogen and hydrogen. Because these are natural penetrating gases, as long as the lungs continue to function freely, one receives the required amount without any material effort. When combined, these gases help to produce the moisture for lung expansion.

It is possible to find more than the listed thirty-six acids in the human body, especially if one takes into account the acids that are detrimental to the human system: the body also contains acids which are created by dead gas in the system, which are dangerous and detrimental to a person's long-term health. I would suggest that as a guideline, a certain portion of acid is necessary for the human body to carry out its daily functions. To explain how one salt creates a certain acid to break down another acid that is injurious to the human body is too long a story. It is of prime importance that we accept that as long as the body has a sufficient amount of various minerals, equally balanced, the acid condition will take care of itself.

Therefore, to protect our health the initial advice is to watch our food intake. Be cautious of citrus fruits and take Molkosan. Remember my advice on the fresh potato juice, and the remedies Gastronol, Centaurium and vitamin supplements. Lastly, I would draw your attention to the Nature's Best remedy called Betaine Hydrochloride, which assists the maintenance of a correct pH balance in the stomach and is especially useful for those over sixty.

Acute gastritis strikes easily and I know that it is often ignored. Be sensible and have it correctly diagnosed, because it must be understood that by doing so, more serious problems at a later stage may be avoided.

Chapter 5

Duodenal Ulcers

Thinking back to my own experience which I mentioned in the opening chapter, I realise I was fortunate being able to control the ulceration of my duodenal ulcer within a relatively short time. Because of the pressure I had been under, there had been a certain amount of internal bleeding. I selected several natural remedies for my personal use and looked at all the factors that were relevant to controlling the situation. I consciously tried to reduce the stress my work involves and also forced myself to take more time for meals. I spread my mealtimes more sensibly, ate more slowly and chewed my food thoroughly. I made sure that I didn't eat extremely hot or cold food, or anything too spicy. I gave up drinking coffee, and fortunately I have never smoked nor do I drink alcohol. Therefore I had no concessions to make in this area. I ate one or two apples a day, but avoided citrus fruits. Moreover, I took Molkosan in an effort to aid my digestion.

To heal the bleeding, every morning and evening I swallowed a teaspoon of St John's Wort oil, which has excellent healing properties. I also took Petasan, Gastronol and Centaurium. Petasan's main ingredient is *Viscum album*, better known as mistletoe, which is combined with *Petasites officinalis* or butterbur. This remedy is highly recommended for impaired or weak circulation, after infectious illness, and in cases of nutritional deficiencies and a weakened condition. I also decided to take ten drops of Lycopodium D6 three times a day, as I had a distended stomach because of acidity and wind. I wanted to reach the heart of the duodenal ulcer and I was aware that because of the tension, the increased hydrochloric acid had caused much damage to the tissue cells. I believe that St John's Wort was the most important factor in my recovery. This herb has such remarkable properties and on many of my visits to the north of Scotland I have heard it praised by members of the older generations, who are very knowledgeable about its potent remedial characteristics.

The pain in my stomach cleared up and my swollen and distended abdomen soon decreased considerably, while the acidity also became less obvious. Of course, overcoming the symptoms was not all I had in mind – I wanted to get to the root of the problem and heal the actual ulcer. Here Gastronol came into its own and three times a day I took five tablets. The intestinal gases were quickly overcome with charcoal tablets.

Now, having told you about my experiences, let's look more generally at stomach ulcers and the resulting acidity. Firstly, I realised that my biggest mistake was that I had not allowed sufficient time for meals because I was too busy. I know from many of my patients that this is a very common occurence. It should be remembered that the digestive process undergoes its first stage of absorption in the mouth. Even our lips have a part to play here. Their thin outer membranes cover an enormous number of blood vessels, giving the lips their red colour. The movement of food around the mouth, which needs chewing again and again, is a vitally important process where tongue, jaws, muscles and cheeks are all involved. The movement of the jaws during the chewing of food is as important as the first stage of the digestion process.

Now we come to the teeth. The last time I travelled to the USA I visited a number of health food stores where the most frequent question I was asked concerned the benefits of fruit and vegetable juices. I was taken aback by the number of questions in this field, but it was explained to me that very recently a gentleman had strongly advocated these raw juices on radio and television. I am certainly not averse to the use of raw fruit and vegetable juices, but I said I was more in favour of strong and healthy teeth. Nature has supplied us with a good set of teeth and in order to stay strong and healthy, they should be used. Raw juices contain beneficial vitamins and minerals, but in taking these foods we are not using our teeth. Juices are fine when circumstances are such that the fresh product is not available, or when physical conditions prevent the use of fresh fruit and vegetables. However, juices are no substitute for the real thing unless there is a very good reason. Take care of your teeth and they may last you a lifetime, which is what they were designed for.

For efficient digestion, the chewing of food is essential in order to increase the production of enzymes in the saliva. Saliva is a sticky substance made up of 90 per cent of water and rich in enzymes. The most important enzyme is amylase. The small amounts of saliva that are secreted in the mouth when eating contain an anti-bacterial action. This helps to prevent the common problem of dental or oral infection. The likelihood of infection is one of the reasons why we ought to inhale through the nose, since by doing so the air intake is filtered. During my years at primary school, tuberculosis was unfortunately common. Our headmaster would visit each classroom every day and drum it into us that we must always breathe in through the nose.

Food is sometimes described as mouthwatering and it is really quite something to realise that sight, smell and even the thought of food increases the flow of saliva in our mouth. The salivary glands are stimulated by both sympathetic and para-sympathetic nerves. Stimulation of the para-sympathetic nerves results in an increase of the blood flow, while stimulation of the sympathetic nerves causes the blood flow to reduce. As much as two and a half pints of saliva are secreted each day, and its function is to maintain the level of acidity in the mouth so that the enzymes can be effective. These facts may make us more appreciative when we sit down for a meal. Thanks to today's social conditions, very few of us know or remember what it is like to be really hungry. The unfortunate outcome of this abundance is that we take our food for granted and we eat without proper enjoyment and attention.

The main ingredients of saliva are glycoprotein, mucin, which gives the saliva its lubricating properties, the enzyme ptyalin which breaks down starch, and lysozine which destroys bacteria. There are also enzymes that dissolve gases and again this process is levelled out by some minerals. It is essential that these substances are mixed well with food, chewed and moistened so that the swallowed food is prepared for the next stage of digestion.

Swallowing involves quite a few muscles that are controlled by the motor nerves. The whole area, even the tongue, the trachea and the nose, are involved in the process of digestion. This process involves all the activities of the digestive tracts and from the very start it depends on correct stimulation. The nutrients from proteins, carbohydrates, fats, salts, vitamins, minerals and trace elements are essential for good health. With the risk of repeating myself, I cannot stress sufficiently that food and its process of digestion starts in the mouth and ends at the rectum. The digestion should be allowed to do its job without interference, and an endoscopy will clearly identify a black area where this process suffers from interference.

The oesophagus is a muscular tube with special rings of muscles known as sphincters, enabling it to open and close at either end. This is where my own problems had originated, because persistent tension had caused a disturbance in the usual process. The wave of muscular contraction known as peristalsis, which is the basis of the movement of food in the entire digestive tract, was severely impaired because it was unable to cope with the speed with which I ate my food, and also with tension caused by my busy lifestyle. The small portion of the smooth muscle of the oesophagus can raise pressure if this tension is too great and can then cause stomach wind and burping as a warning.

Acting as a storehouse for ingested food is one of the stomach's important functions. For this process to work correctly we depend to a large extent on a healthy and regular bowel movement. The waste residue of any ingested food should be able to leave the body unhindered, in order to avoid problems such as I had experienced.

So often we hear that a friend or acquaintance has an ulcer, and whether this is a duodenal or a gastric ulcer, we must remember that it is a painful affliction. I well remember the days when, in the middle of a busy surgery, I would feel the onset of a rhythmic periodic pain, which either remained as a dull ache or discomfort, or developed into sharp and severe spasmodic pain. The pain caused by a duodenal ulcer is located in the right epigastrium under the sternum and is expressed in sharp spasms. Sometimes it relents when something is eaten, but that chronic, recurring, penetrating pain with a nauseous sensation is something I never want to experience again. From personal experience I would emphasise that when the first alarm bells start ringing, please do something positive about it. Remember that although the first indication may only be flatulence, excessive burping or a feeling of discomfort could soon develop into a more serious condition if it is allowed to continue unchecked.

Reaching a correct diagnosis may not be so simple without an endoscopy, but with a gastric or duodenal ulcer the first signs are spasms of pain, irritability and tenderness. Drinking the juice of raw potatoes, cabbage or carrots, especially if these juices are taken as part of a wholesome diet, may well help to overcome such a condition.

Although I have already given some dietary advice in the opening chapter, a special diet is important for the first stages of a threatened ulcer. Before breakfast take a half glass of raw potato juice diluted with warm water. Breakfast should consist of wholewheat which has been soaked in water for two or three days. It can be made more palatable with a good vegetable stock or fresh butter. Crispbread with butter and wheatgerm should complete the breakfast, according to Dr Vogel. If the bowels require special attention, take some freshly ground linseed, always remembering that it must be chewed very thoroughly. The liver will benefit from raw carrot juice. For lunch have a healthy vegetable soup with a quarter-pint of raw cabbage juice added and have some fresh vegetables or a salad. For the salad dressing use Molkosan instead of vinegar.

People who are very nervous and tired will benefit from a raw egg beaten with a little grape juice, which also serves as a good blood-former. Do not cook the egg, because most of its vitamins will be destroyed and uric acid will increase. A raw egg is curative in any diet. Supper can be the same as breakfast, or you may prefer a plate of porridge. Although I stated earlier that eating fresh fruit is preferable to simply drinking its juice, in this case it is better to drink the fresh juice extracted from the fruit. A fresh soup with plenty of vegetables, a thick minestrone for example, is very beneficial.

I must also remind you that fruit and vegetables should never be eaten together. Reserve fruit for one meal and vegetables for another, and allow some time in between. Note also that bananas and melons should always be eaten separately as these are so-called 'jealous' foods that do not mix well. I am often asked why fruit and vegetables should not be mixed, and the reason is that it can cause problems for the digestion. It is not good either to drink juices when they are too cold. When he discovered that ice cubes had been added to his fruit juice, I once heard Dr Vogel remonstrate that he was not born in Alaska. He is quite right: to bombard the stomach with these icy cold juices is not helpful. The acids of the juices are not always well tolerated, and it is much better to sip them slowly. The gastric mucous membranes are sensitive and deserve consideration.

Whilst preparing this section I saw an old farmer who has been a patient at the clinic for quite some time. At one time he told me that his doctor had warned him about a threatened ulcer, and knowing that he had plenty of cabbages on his farm, I asked him to try and drink half a pint of fresh cabbage juice a day. It can be combined with carrot juice to make it more palatable. Since then he has told me that the condition was now completely under control. Just because these are old remedies does not mean they are less effective. I have also seen ulcers brought under control with the use of clay powder. With the help of nature many problems can be eliminated, but only if we follow a well-balanced diet. This, together with one or more remedies, relaxation exercises and herbal remedies, can make all the difference.

Chapter 6

Gastric Ulcers

The origins of duodenal and gastric ulcers are fundamentally different. A lack of mucosal protection is often the cause of a duodenal ulcer, whereas a combination of irritation and inflammation of the stomach lining is largely the cause of gastric ulceration. The lack of a healthy blood supply to the area also plays a big part, as this of course has a healing effect. Furthermore, whilst the duodenal ulcer is mostly caused by an imbalance of acid and peptic enzymes, the gastric ulcer is caused by a variety of reasons. In the case of a duodenal ulcer some relief may be obtained from eating, but this action will only aggravate a gastric ulcer.

Indigestion and heartburn usually affect the acid stomach secretions, which then cause a gastric condition. The average adult secretes a considerable amount of gastric juice, but much depends on the quality of these juices. Over-acidity, flatulence and abdominal distension due to wind denote a duodenal ulcer, with accompanying stomach pain. In the case of a gastric ulcer the tendency is towards vomiting, haemorrhage or even blood-coloured stools. I have come to the conclusion that the cause of gastric ulcers is slightly different. Over-eating is definitely one reason, and the use of aluminium cooking pots is also a possibility. Excess sugar consumption and vitamin and mineral deficiencies are also held to be responsible. A shortage of the vitamins A, B and C, and calcium in particular, is rather common.

To combat the effects of over-acidity for people with a gastric ulcer, I mostly advise them to take Gastronol together with

Urticalcin and also a vitamin supplement. For the latter I usually suggest Health Insurance Plus from Nature's Best, which combines thirty-four nutrients into a single convenient tablet. This remedy is chosen by many health practitioners who appreciate the reliability of an all-round supplement that will not interfere with a patient's effort to maintain health. Many supplements cannot be used by people whose vitality is low and who may be sensitive to ingredients that are used as the base for concentrated nutrients. In line with the latest research into allergies and sensitivities, Nature's Best has developed a 'hypo-allergenic' base for Health Insurance Plus, using only those ingredients to which allergic people are least likely to react. It is guaranteed free from wheat, grains, soya, corn, yeast (important especially for people being treated for Candida albicans), dairy products and salicylates. It almost goes without saying that artificial colours, preservatives, sugar and flavourings are also excluded. Health Insurance Plus is therefore ideal for anyone planning to protect their nutritional status by taking a multi-supplement regularly over a long period of time. The following list shows the formidable supplement of vitamins, minerals and trace elements that each tablet contains:

Vitamin A	1120iu
Vitamin D3	23iu
Vitamin B1	11.5mg
Vitamin B2	6mg
Vitamin B6	14mg
Vitamin B12	25mcg
Vitamin C	134mg
Vitamin E d-alpha toc. succinate	45iu
Biotin	34mcg
Calcium Pantothenate (B5)	57mg
Choline (as Bitartrate)	11.5mg
Lemon Bioflavenoids	22mg
Folic Acid	67mcg
Nicotinic Acid	9mg
Nicotinamide	17mg
Inositol	11.5mg
PABA	6mg
Beta Carotene	4mg

Iodine (as Potassium Iodide)	23mcg
Calcium (Oyster shell fine micronised)	110mg
Chromium (as Orotate)	22mcg
Iron (as Fumarate)	2.68mcg
Magnesium Aspartate	56mg
Magnesium (as Oxide)	56mg
Manganese (as Orotate)	2mg
Molybdenum (as Potassium Molybdate)	12mcg
Potassium Aspartate	17mg
Selenium (as Seleno-L-Merhionine)	22mcg
Zinc (as Gluconate)	3.5mg
L-Cyestine	28mg
Glycine	3mg
Glutamic Acid	3.5mg
L-Methionine	1.35mg

I especially like the inclusion of minerals and trace elements in this combination supplement, as these substances are often very beneficial for peptic ulcers. Sometimes this can give surprising results as I again witnessed recently with a patient who had been unsuccessful with the prescribed orthodox medical treatment. This patient told me that digestive disorders were very common in his family, and people often enquire if digestive or ulcer problems are hereditary. Certainly this tendency is often the case, and quite often I recognise a nervous or sensitive trait in the background of certain families. It also depends greatly on a mother's lifestyle during pregnancy. One of my greatest worries is alcohol, as this breaks down the single enzyme dehydrogenase or ADH in the foetus. When the liver breaks down alcohol, ADH is formed, and can cause an upset stomach which in turn can be the cause of stomach ulcers. Not only is this very uncomfortable for the pregnant mother, but there is also the risk that this may affect the unborn baby. Disorders of the pancreas, malnutrition, or injury to the liver could result and therefore alcohol should be avoided. The same applies to nicotine.

Gastric ulcers produce pain and discomfort within thirty minutes of eating. These are fairly quickly diagnosed and should have immediate attention. Although peptic ulcers may be associated with certain blood groups, with gastric ulcers the likelihood of this is not so strong. People with blood group A are slightly more susceptible to gastric ulcers than those with blood group O, which is linked to an over-production of cells. People with blood group B seem to be more prone to duodenal ulcers. Very often aspirin is taken for the pain, but this is unwise because this analgesic can actually be the cause of ulcers and could well result in perforation. Aspirin inhibits the production of prostaglandins, and because this substance protects the lining of the stomach, drugs such as aspirin may aggravate the situation.

One difference between duodenal and gastric ulcers is that the latter are more common in the elderly, while the former are more likely to occur in younger people. Also it seems that duodenal ulcers are more prevalent among males, while gastric ulcers occur irrespective of gender. Food aggravates gastric ulcers, though it is not known whether it has any influence on duodenal ulcers. People with the blood group O are more easily affected by duodenal ulcers, while those with blood group A are more subject to gastric ulcers. Nausea and vomiting are less common with duodenal ulcers than with gastric ulcers, which have wind and burping as symptoms instead. Duodenal ulcers also result in more acidity than gastric ulcers. These are just a few differences between the two types of ulcers.

I always feel sorry when people with a gastric ulcer consent to surgery. During the operation a branch of the vagus nerve is removed in an attempt to moderate the flow of acid to the stomach, so allowing the ulcer to heal. But there are many remedies that enable patients to overcome a gastric ulcer without surgery. In the first place the body must rid itself of the underlying acidity, but this is not done by neutralisation with alkaline chemicals. It makes sense to explore what can be achieved with dietary changes, and for this purpose it is useful to follow the diet guidelines in the first chapter. Sometimes a fast can be beneficial, or a full milk diet for three to six days. Take as much rest as possible and then gradually start eating solids, such as stewed fruit, which is gentler on the stomach than fresh fruit. Avoid citrus fruits, spices, coffee, tea and any pork products. Eat live yoghurt, perhaps with stewed fruit, as well as cooked vegetables and cottage cheese. This is gentler and better than a diet of fresh fruit and vegetables. On the subject of bowel cleansing, it must be understood that there should be no constipation. See Chapter 14 for more advice on that specific subject. Fresh air and gentle relaxation exercises are important and I would suggest some gentle osteopathic manipulation if possible.

On my many visits to the USA I often come across patients with ulcer problems. I am inclined to believe that ulcers are more prevalent there because of a general tendency in Americans to over-eat. The best general advice I can give is to stop eating at the point where food still tastes at its best. Anything eaten after that moment tends to be stored as fat and it is widely accepted that over-eating has a strong bearing on stomach problems. The intricate digestive process works so efficiently if we allow it to do its job unhindered. We should do everything possible to allow that system to do what it does best.

I have already mentioned that fasting can be helpful, and some people try to fast one day a week. This makes good sense as it gives the stomach a brief respite on a regular basis. Another idea is to substitute all food with fruit juice at mealtimes and you will feel mentally and physically invigorated. Single-day fasts are not too rigorous on the system, but a three-day fast should be conducted under the correct conditions only. You must make sure that you are able to rest at convenient times during the day. Completely relax by avoiding company, television, radio and reading. Retire to your bedroom and remain there for most of the fast. This régime has worked very well in our clinics. On fasting days there we often mention the importance of bed rest, because at these times detoxification and internal cleansing take place. Have a short walk outdoors periodically and for the remainder of the time complete rest. We should be aware of the pressure placed on our stomach by everyday tensions. It is noticeable that under these conditions weight loss is much more considerable than strenuous physical exercise could produce. It is possible to feel a little light-headed, but this can easily be overcome by relaxing.

People are very concerned about the functioning of their bowels during a period of fasting. It is possible that bowel movement may stop all together, but there is no need to worry because this will adjust itself when the fast ends. Do not force the issue by using enemas or bowel irrigation, but instead let nature take its course. After a fast be careful how you reintroduce solids to the diet. Take light food, such as cooked vegetables and fruit, but be wary of dairy products, meat and fish. A few pieces of toast are helpful and in general it is best to choose some easily digested food. Remember that apples, bananas or pineapple contain good digestive enzymes, but always eat these separately. For example, if you have decided to follow a diet of bananas, never mix them with other fruits. In its own way a banana has a similar effect to milk whey or sour milk, providing a better bacterial balance in the body. For people with colitis, abdominal and bowel disorders, bananas are a valuable non-irritant food. I am well aware that this fruit is often criticised, but I can assure you that it can be taken without danger.

To repeat what has already been stated, yoghurt is very beneficial, especially the plain variety without added flavour or fruit. If you so desire you can add a mashed banana or some honey. There is so much natural protein in yoghurt, and its calcium, phosphorus, vitamin A, riboflavin and niacin content make it into an excellent and healthy dessert. It also lowers the blood alcohol level and helps digestion. Yoghurt made from goat's milk is easier to digest than that made from cow's milk. For a tasty treat, try a yoghurt made from sheep's milk; the only drawback is that its fat content is much higher and therefore it should not be eaten too often or in great quantities. Remember the rule that diet must be kept as natural as possible.

The treatment of a gastric ulcer must be taken seriously, in case it develops into a carcinogenic situation. Take Gastronol, charcoal tablets and Petasan. Unless there is bleeding, the latter has great healing properties. In the case of a bleeding ulcer, however, I would suggest that the patient takes witch-hazel (*Hamamelis virginiana*). Petasan has great healing properties for all kinds of ulcer problems, but is also a great cell-renewer. If it is administered in the right dosage, together with *Viscum album*, patients benefit greatly. *Viscum album*, or mistletoe, is an extra-ordinary plant which, unlike other plants, grows downwards rather than upwards. Nature may have sent us a coded message: the plant is active and wants to restore. Extraordinarily, mistletoe grows like a parasite – not unlike a cancer would grow in the body – yet it is there to balance and heal and restore health.

Chapter 7

Pancreatitis

The pancreas is an organ which is situated behind and just below the stomach and it is an important source of digestive juices. Each day the pancreas produces 1,200 to 1,500cc (about two and a half pints) of clear liquid called pancreatic juice, which pours down to the pancreatic duct. When food enters through the mouth the taste-buds send impulses to the brain, which responds by stimulating the pancreas through the vagus nerve. Two hormones are secreted, pancreozymin and secretin, both of which stimulate the production of pancreatic juices. These juices contain several enzymes, but the main three are as follows:

- lipase, which is the only fat-digesting enzyme;
- amylase, for the digestion of carbohydrates;
- trypsin inhibitor, which prevents the pancreatic juices becoming active until they have reached the duodenum, otherwise they would digest the pancreas itself.

Apart from the digestive function, the pancreas produces essential hormones such as insulin and glucagon from the group of cells which are known as the Islets of Langerhans. Glucagon accelerates the conversion of glucogen to glucose. Insulin on the other hand opposes glucagon, decreasing the blood-sugar level by accelerating the transportation of glucose into the cells. The working of these two hormones control the body's energy. In other words, the pancreas controls a tremendous number of our body functions. It is therefore very important that we look after it to the best of our ability. We see that this is often not the case if we examine the many problems of high and low blood-sugar, in other words diabetes and hypoglycaemia. However, in this chapter I want to concentrate on pancreatitis, because over the years I have seen quite a few cases among my patients.

Pancreatitis is the name given to a condition which is mostly marked by an inflammation of the pancreas. When it occurs in an acute state it is associated with inflammation and necrosis of the adjacent omentum and viscera, with or without haemorrhage. There is also chronic interstitial pancreatitis which is an inflammation, usually non-specific, causing a gradual replacement of the parenchyna by fibrosis. Although this condition is not very common, immediate steps must be taken when it occurs. The inflammation, which is very often attributed to the regurgitation of bile from the common bile duct into the major pancreatic duct, is a situation which can cause tremendous pain. Other symptoms are severe nausea, vomiting, spasms, tachycardia, tenderness, and so on. It is said that 75 per cent of all cases are due to biliary tract disease, sometimes caused by calculi in the duct, or cholecystitis.

It is very often found by enzyme studies in cases of pancreatitis that an inflammation in the glands can lead to a perforated ulcer, acute cholecystitis and appendicitis. In its early stage it may be a pancreatic abscess and especially with cases of chronic pancreatitis careful action should be taken. Very mild cases, which are fairly general, will respond to remedies and rest, especially bed rest and a special diet. Chronic interstitial pancreatitis can cause very acute attacks and usually the symptoms are fatty and bulky stools, owing to pancreatic deficiencies. Very often jaundice is involved. It must be said that chronic pancreatitis is often incorrectly diagnosed and that the mortality rate of sufferers is unfortunately quite high. Specialised care is essential.

We often see that in an unbalanced acid-alkaline diet the pancreatic fluid is not efficient in digesting the partly digested proteins and starches present in the food. Often, after eating too much, little cramps can remind us that the pancreas is not working the way it should, and if this happens, a hot shower on the stomach for ten to fifteen minutes can relieve that uncomfortable feeling.

We must not forget that the pancreas, along with the liver, is one of the most important organs in the body. Although the liver is twenty times heavier than the pancreas, this little gland, which is so important in the whole endocrine system, plays an enormous role. If we think of the phenomenal biochemical functions that this gland fulfils in influencing all the other organs of the body, we realise that we must treat it with respect – something which, unfortunately, the majority of people do not do.

Several times already in this book I have mentioned the remedy called Molkosan. This liquid was the inspiration of Dr Vogel. It occurred to him when he thought about the process of manufacturing cheese, that the milk whey, which is the residue, was thrown away. This milk acid, which is produced by a natural fermentation process which conserves all the nutrients and minerals, is rich in natural dextrorotatory lactic acid. This makes it a wonderful remedy for patients with Candida albicans.

More than three litres of whey are required to produce one litre of Molkosan. Not only is Molkosan a terrific antiseptic, but it also assists in balancing the bacteria in the large intestine and aids the digestive system. Because the acid is right-turning (dextrorotatory) it will also produce extra oxygen in the cells. A left-turning milk acid cannot be broken down, so it is important that Molkosan is taken as a remedy which also produces natural insulin.

I advise every diabetic patient to take this on a daily basis and I have seen a wonderful improvement in patients who were on insulin, able to control their diabetes by taking tablets and later by a healthy natural diet and some herbal remedies.

This regulating mechanism ensures that the correct percentage of glucose is always present. This is necessary for glycogen which is stored in the liver and some muscles. The circulating glucose and the glucose content of the blood, known as the blood-sugar mirror, must be kept at the right level. The Islets of Langerhans cells in the pancreas secrete insulin. Basically the action of insulin increases the rate of glucose transfer through the cell membrane. When the blood-glucose level rises, the pancreas automatically secretes insulin. The insulin causes the surplus glucose to be stored as glycogen in the cells. When the blood-sugar level is too low, the pancreas pours glucagon into the bloodstream. In turn, the glucagon stimulates the almost immediate release of glucose from the liver, thus causing the blood-sugar level to rise. When the pancreas is healthy and everything is working well, blood-sugar levels are maintained within acceptable limits. If, however, the pancreas produces too little or too much insulin, then correction is necessary. It is therefore essential to use some remedies if there is the slightest imbalance, one of the very best of which is the walnut. I have found that in both diabetes and hypoglycaemia, walnuts have produced terrific results.

I have often wondered about the true meaning of the word 'science'. I think that the best definition is: discovering the secrets of nature and making these available to man. Unfortunately in this day and age we have forgotten this. On the inside of the walnut there is a paper-thin tissue – let us call it the membrane – which has ingredients which are so beneficial for the pancreas. My mother was diabetic and managed to control her condition very well. She used to buy two pounds of walnuts every week. She used the nuts in her salads, but instead of discarding the shells, she would boil them with the membranes still inside. To one pound of walnuts she added two pints of water, boiled it and drank a cupful a day, while she stored the rest in the fridge for the following days. This is one of the finest remedies for the pancreas. Pineapple or blackcurrant juice, herbal juices and fasting are other excellent ways of helping the pancreas. This is much better, especially with an acute pancreatitis, than to take alcohol, spices, nicotine, or develop metabolic disturbances through an over-consumption of sugary or fatty foods. With an imbalanced food pattern, gallstones may be produced which can cause pancreatic irritation. Even when the pancreas is damaged there can be a tremendous improvement in absorption through taking the correct nutrition.

When there has been an infection it is beneficial to use the natural antibiotic Echinaforce. Over the years this has proved to be a great help in cases of inflammation and infection as well as in special cases of acute pancreatitis. To keep the pancreas healthy when there is a sensitivity or a possible dysfunction, the remedy Pancreatin from Nature's Best is of great benefit. Pancreatin contains:

Lipase	5,200 units
Protease	32,500 units
Amylase	32,500 units

The leaflets accompanying Nature's Best products explain that enzymes contribute to the functioning of the numerous processes within the body. Indeed, many vitamins are often referred to as co-enzymes because they are used by the body in its countless metabolic pathways only in conjunction with enzymes. Digestive enzymes are used by the body to release from food all vitamins and minerals which are needed for good health.

The three main digestive enzymes each work on a different type of food in order to prepare it for digestion. Protease breaks down protein, amylase breaks down starch and lipase breaks down fats. Like all enzymes in the body they act as catalysts, which means they promote and speed up chemical reactions without becoming part of them. Usually when all these intricate functions are working in a healthy balance, we can prevent the problems on which I will concentrate in the following chapters.

Chapter 8

Gastroenteritis and Food Poisoning

Gastroenteritis is an acute inflammation of the lining of the stomach and the intestines. At one time it was thought to be caused by alcohol, or food and drink poisoning, induced by drugs or, even worse, by heavy metals. The severity of this problem depends totally upon what has been swallowed. Usually the first signs are nausea, abdominal cramps, diarrhoea, flu symptoms, a distended abdomen and intestinal wind. It is usually easily diagnosed by its symptoms, but in more severe cases a sigmoidoscopy may be needed. Fast action must be taken, and food poisoning is more common nowadays than ever.

There are various strains of gastroenteritis, such as chronic enteritis or food poisoning, which is often caused by ingesting food that has been contaminated by certain bacteria. When the liver becomes impaired hospitalisation can be necessary. However, non-bacterial food poisoning can be due to many different causes, among them mushroom or mussel poisoning, metal contaminants or sometimes enamel poisoning. What we should always consider is food safety: it is the key to good health. Food must be stored under the correct conditions, whether it be fresh, preserved, tinned or in a frozen state. I have often seen food poisoning symptoms caused by 'E numbers' or additives, to which the patient has had an allergic reaction.

A while ago I had a case which puzzled me for quite some time. The patient who faced me across the desk was very off colour and although food poisoning was obvious, I could not identify the offending factor. Like a detective I questioned her on all the different possibilities, but every time we drew a blank. Then suddenly the penny dropped. She mentioned in passing that her freezer, which mostly contained meat and fish, had had its electricity supply cut off for over twenty-four hours. When the power was eventually restored, she re-froze the contents. With this bit of information I knew that there was no need to look further for the source of contamination.

It should be remembered that guidelines for food storage have been developed for the consumer's benefit. It is not a matter of red tape or bureaucrats meddling in affairs that are not their concern. The fact is that correct storage methods for food can make the difference between good and poor health. Whether it be fresh or frozen food, it must be stored and cooked properly. To my sorrow I often notice that all too often frozen food is first of all defrosted, and then cooked in a microwave oven. Always read the labels on the packaging carefully to check on the ingredients used and to look for preparation instructions.

Bacteria, depending on the strain, can have either a positive or a negative effect, but in order to reduce the risk of food poisoning the highest standards of hygiene must be maintained. It is very encouraging that one of the aims of the World Health Organisation is to advise on ways of avoiding or minimising the risks of food poisoning. The final responsibility is ours, however. Occasionally I do a spot of shopping and nip into a supermarket or a corner-shop. Sometimes I see soiled and damaged packaging and dented tins on the shelves. I would never buy these products and I suggest that the retailer removes these items from the shelves. It is a great bonus for the consumer that the shelf-life of many food products has now been officially established and that this is displayed as a 'sell by' date. It only requires a little common sense to know that when you have bought frozen foods, you do not deposit them in the car and continue with the rest of your shopping. No, you do your shopping first and then, to minimise the risk of defrosting, you drive home immediately with your frozen food and store it safely in the freezer. Make sure that the temperature in your freezer or refrigerator is correct, because bacterial invaders can multiply very quickly. Hygiene and cleanliness must be observed and animals should always be kept away from food.

Not so long ago a major outbreak of salmonella poisoning was responsible for the death of a number of elderly patients in a nursing home. At the inquest some light was shed on the matter. The nursing home used to obtain their weekly egg deliveries from a specific supplier whose hygiene standards were closely monitored. However, another supplier quoted a more competitive price for their regular deliveries and this new supplier won the contract. Apparently raw eggs had been used in the preparation of mayonnaise and ice-cream, and these raw eggs were discovered to be the source of the infection which had spread rampantly through the residents of the nursing home. How sad that so much unnecessary pain and suffering was the result of what was actually no more than an economic decision. It was hardly fair to put all the blame on the chef, who himself had contracted hepatitis. When he attended our clinic for treatment we talked at length about the unfortunate affair. Fortunately, he responded well to the Bioforce remedy Boldo-cynara for liver and biliary problems. This fresh herb preparation stimulates bile production, and is especially de-signed for the treatment of liver insufficiency, disturbances in the metabolic rate, digestive insufficiencies, dyskinesia of the liver and bile passages. I often prescribe this remedy for food poisoning cases, sometimes together with charcoal and Nux Vomica D-4. If diarrhoea is one of the symptoms, I recommend that the patient also takes Tormentavena, which quickly re-duces inflammation of the mucous membranes of the intestinal tract and bleeding haemorrhoids. This remedy contains the following ingredients:

Potentilla erecta	Tormentil
Lythrum salicaria	Loosestrife
Galeopsis ochr.	Hemp nettle
Polygonum aviculare	Knotweed
Avena sativa	Oats
Petasites officinalis	Butterbur

These are excellent remedies for the treatment of hepatitis and luckily the chef recovered quickly. Unfortunately some of the nursing home patients did not have the same chance, especially as many of them were elderly and moreover weakened by the condition for which they had been taken into the nursing home in the first place.

Another warning to heed concerns some of the more exotic cheeses that are available nowadays. The milk used for quite a few of these cheeses is non-pasteurised and could irritate the stomachs of the very young and the elderly.

There is also concern about the practice of reheating food. Repeated reheating does not enhance quality and I was quite horrified when I recently read in a newspaper that 45,000 cases of food poisoning had been reported in one year. The report made it clear that it was not just salmonella and lysteria which usually make it into the headlines, but also other more common bacteria which caused problems.

While on the subject of cooking I must take this opportunity to share with you my concern about the increased use of microwave ovens. I have stated several times already how important it is to keep our food as natural as possible and, to my way of thinking, cooking food in a microwave oven must fall outside this category. This point is stressed in my book *Nature's Gift of Food*.

Time and again it amazes me when I see how many people leave public conveniences without washing their hands. By doing so, they endanger not only their own health, but also the health of others. It is so important from the point of view of hygiene that we wash our hands regularly, and toilets and kitchens must be kept clean. Too many people have had cause to regret that they overlooked or underrated what they considered a minor point of hygiene. If we are lucky we can get away with it once or twice, or possibly even a few more times, but once misfortune has struck, it is too late.

On one of my transatlantic journeys I arrived desperately ill at my destination. For three days I was unable to leave my bed and there was no doubt that I had contracted a severe case of food poisoning. I can only think that the food on board the aircraft was somehow contaminated. Fortunately, I have a strong constitution and therefore this was a most unusual experience for me. Whatever remedies I took, I had to allow them to take their course, and this was my first, and thank goodness only, experience of gastroenteritis. This personal experience has certainly encouraged a sympathetic understanding towards my patients who are struck by food poisoning.

With a bout of food poisoning immediate fasting is often beneficial. Take plenty of fluids and stay in bed, after which light and easily digested food can be gradually reintroduced. If a baby suffers food poisoning a few drops of Echinaforce will help quickly. This is my favourite natural remedy because of its antibiotic properties. Strawberry leaf tea or strawberry extract is also often very helpful for the very young.

Patients sometimes tell me that they have not felt too well since they ate this, that or the other dish. I once overheard two ladies in conversation in a restaurant after they finished their lunch, and one of them claimed not to feel very well. With a serious look on her face she told her friend that she had not enjoyed her meal, but as she had paid for it, she felt obliged to eat and finish it. It does not make sense, does it? Never eat unsafe food, even if there is only the slightest doubt.

Food can be contaminated in more ways than one; it is not only eggs or exotic cheeses which can cause problems, but also unpasteurised milk, mouldy or unripe food, and only too often fruit that has not been washed properly. So often vegetables have been sprayed with herbicides or pesticides and unless this is washed off very thoroughly, adverse reactions when they are eaten are more than likely. Of course it is advisable to eat the skin of most fruit, but always wash them well.

One other piece of advice is that not all bottled water is as safe as one might imagine it to be. Choose a brand which you know well, preferably in a glass bottle rather than a plastic container. Sometimes bottled water is allowed to stay on the shop shelves for so long that bacteria develops or becomes active, and this is more likely to happen in plastic containers. The same applies to ice cubes and iced drinks, of course.

Whilst travelling through Far Eastern countries I have often come across problems resulting from uncooked seafood. Another time, when I worked in a hospital in India, I asked my colleague if the large number of patients seeking treatment for minor and major stomach upsets was unusual (in a hot country bacteria develop very much more quickly than in our more temperate climate). I was told that in recent years food hygiene in India had much improved. It was accepted though, that food poisoning was a recurring problem because of the climate.

If I learn that patients of mine are planning to go away on holiday to certain countries, I advise them to pack Echinaforce, Gastronol and charcoal tablets. Every traveller can take the same precautions and for many it means the difference between a successful or a ruined holiday.

I knew a fisherman from the north of Scotland. He was most flattered to be invited to help in the development of the fishing industry of Ghana. When he told me about his project in Africa I was fascinated and wished him good luck. Two months later when I saw him again I hardly recognised him: he was a physical wreck because he had been plagued intermittently by gastroenteritis. He had become exposed to some unidentified viral activity, and in fact several people expressed doubt that he would survive. He was transported back to Scotland in a very serious condition, and when I saw him I realised that we had a lot of work to do to reverse his condition. He put his faith in me and followed my advice. With fasting, herbal and homoeopathic remedies, we managed to pull him through. Later, when he was asked to return to Ghana to take up the reins of the project again, he suggested that they would be wiser to contract a younger person, because he dared not risk his health again.

If there is a problem, always attend to it quickly and remember the adage, prevention is better than cure. Remember also that food is necessary to man for energy. By ignoring hygiene requirements, especially in food preparation, it is easy to destroy the nutritional value and the quality of food. Always keep food as natural as possible so that what we eat brings life, not death.

Chapter 9

Appendicitis and Peritonitis

Some time ago the case of a good friend of mine received a great deal of attention from an eminent medical specialist and I was rather taken aback by some of the observations which were made. This friend had an incurable disease and it was obvious that he did not have long to live. However, he never gave up hope, did everything he was asked and explored every possibility. This was why he made an appointment to see this specialist. This doctor examined my friend in my presence and eventually said that if the patient still had his appendix he might have been able to do some more for him. I was greatly intrigued and asked him for an explanation, but unfortunately just at that moment he was called away and I never met him again.

Later I heard it confirmed from various sources that in the case of degenerative disease the appendix appears to have a certain function that may actually help the condition. This confirms my long-standing belief that every part of the body, no matter how small, has a function. It is quite likely that the specialist was correct in his assumption, which saddens me even more when I consider how often an appendix is removed, without this operation being absolutely necessary. Please do not misunderstand me: I am not suggesting that an appendix should never be removed under any circumstances; if it is inflamed it must be removed. However, sometimes this is done without the firm knowledge that the appendix is the source of the patient's problem. We cannot just remove organs at random, even though it is believed that removal of a particular organ will not impair the body's function, but will rather eliminate a possible problem.

Appendicitis is an inflammation of the vermiform appendix and surgery is essential in cases of perforation. I have treated many 'grumbling appendices' in my career and I have seen many patients who would have been operated on by a conventional doctor. These patients have escaped the knife because there are ways of avoiding surgery, unless the inflammation has spread too far. Much can be done to help a grumbling appendix and the remedy Hyperisan has been used by many people as an alternative to surgery. This remedy also belongs to the Bioforce range and contains the following:

Achillea millefolium	Yarrow
Aesculus hipp.	Horse chestnut
Hypericum perforatum	St John's Wort
Arnica montana e radix	Arnica herb and root

Appendicitis causes pain in the epigastric region, and is sometimes symptomised by vomiting and tenderness. Acute appendicitis is often associated with a high fever, and the correct diagnosis is essential. When the appendix becomes inflamed or infected, the opening between the caecum and the appendix becomes blocked. Appendicitis can be related to many things, often to constipation, a low-fibre diet, or other deficiencies which can cause the organ to become inflamed. With a sensible diet the condition may still be reversed. Never wait until the appendix perforates, however, because by then there is a very real risk of peritonitis. Always seek medical help immediately and drink small amounts of water, tea or diluted fruit juice, but do not take coffee or alcohol. I have found that taking ten drops of Hyperisan three times a day often eases a grumbling appendix. Kept up for a few days, this is very often sufficient to relieve the condition and allow the body to take over and heal itself.

It is fairly unusual for the appendix to turn sceptic without prior warning. Usually it is the result of a bowel condition which has been toxic for quite some time, and starts to infect the appendix, which is a small organ located at the very beginning of the large intestine. Despite many statements to the contrary, I still believe that the appendix has a role to play in our overall health and this was obviously confirmed by the specialist who attended to my friend.

Avoid constipation, irregular bowel movements, or a toxic bowel condition which may have developed as a result of ingesting toxic material. Too often we see that the removal of the appendix does not improve the general condition of the patient, because in many cases the root of the problem lay elsewhere and this surgery has not touched upon the cause of the infection. Many patients have been spared the experience of a surgical operation for the removal of a grumbling appendix by such simple remedies as fasting.

As the appendix patient is usually nervous and tense at the start of the fast, the effects are often quickly noticeable. The patient must rest and it may be helpful to cover the painful area with hot or chamomile compresses. It is sometimes beneficial to administer a coffee enema or even a hot water enema, which quickly clears the abdominal area. Keep this up for a few days and drink fruit juices in preference to solid food. Try a fruit diet for a full week, and if the constipation is still persistent, I strongly recommend that the patient takes Linoforce. This is a natural laxative, ideal for the purpose of regulating intestinal activity and giving temporary relief from occasional constipation, and increasing the frequency of bowel movements. Linoforce contains the following ingredients:

Semen lini tot.	Flaxseed
Fol. sennae	Senna leaves
Cortex frangulea	Alder buckthorn bark
Calcium lacticum	Calcium
Ol. zingiberia	Ginger oil
Vanilla planifolia	Vanilla

If a patient suffers considerable discomfort, he or she may benefit from a sitz bath to which mustard seed has been added. It is also advisable to drink herbal teas such as chamomile or peppermint tea. Get sufficient rest and sleep and give the appendix a chance to detoxify. This can be aided by what Dr Vogel calls 'The Spring Cleansing Course', which is based on various herbal remedies.

It is now widely believed that infection of the appendix is the result of internal pollution, which can eventually lead to the development of cancerous problems. Carcinogenic substances (that is, cancer-causing substances) affect the immune system, and their paralysing effect on it will allow the gradual (or rampant) growth of a cancer. A fully functioning appendix, which my friend of course lacked, might possibly have benefited his immune system in this very difficult time.

If appendicitis is treated in the natural way, the risk of peritonitis can be virtually ignored. Peritonitis is an acute or chronic inflammation of the peritoneum which lines the abdominal cavity. Perforation of a ruptured appendix, a peptic ulcer, diverticulitis, or invaders such as intestinal parasites, can result in a peritonitis condition. The way this condition manifests itself varies. With a chronic peritonitis the discomfort is likely to be less than in the case of acute peritonitis. Whatever the condition, a natural antibiotic such as Echinaforce and small doses of Petasan should be taken. It is more important with peritonitis that early and adequate treatment is given. Infections of many kinds, intestinal obstructions, or even carcinomas which are unchecked, can complicate the problem.

Perforation can allow partially digested food and bacteria from the digestive tract to enter the abdominal cavity, causing peritonitis and inflammation. Unless immediate action is taken, surgery may be the only option.

Chapter 10

Colitis and Ulcerative Colitis

Ulcerative colitis is an inflammatory disease of the colon that attacks the mucous membrane lining of the large intestine, which comprises the colon and rectum. Colitis upsets the normal function of the lining and it becomes raw, red, inflamed and ulcerated. Sufferers experience attacks of uncontrollable diarrhoea, often with considerable loss of blood and mucus, and sometimes severe abdominal pain.

Colitis is similar to Crohn's disease, but whereas colitis attacks only the colon, Crohn's disease may affect any part of, or even the whole digestive canal. What causes ulcerative colitis and Crohn's disease remains a mystery. Some research has suggested that a fault in the body's immune system could allow damage to the mucous membrane. Other investigations have looked at the possibility that bacteria or a virus could be the culprit. Stress, smoking, diet and environmental factors have also been suggested as possible contributory factors.

Over the years more and more mysterious diseases have been identified that attack the bowel wall, mostly resulting in chronic intestinal inflammation. Inflammatory diseases include conditions such as proctitis, enteritis, colitis, ulcerative colitis, and so on. One might classify colitis as a mucus colitis, while others regard it as the sign of an irritable colon. The differences in colitis problems are many, but if ignored, relatively minor problems could well become aggravated and develop into a chronic ulcerative colitis. This is a non-specific inflammatory ulcerative disease which can lead to much more severe problems.

Colitis can be characterised by frequent watery stools and lower abdominal discomfort, and pains similar to colic pains. The irritated mucous lining of the colon tends to cause a more smelly stool than usual. When this condition is allowed to continue, eventually the stage is reached where drugs are unable to improve the state of the colon and sometimes even a change in the diet may not have much impact on the situation. The whole condition must be taken into consideration and the cause of the colitis must be located. This can be different in every patient.

When a person becomes concerned and anxious, this stress can block the sympathetic nerve plexus, while there is a secretion of excessive adrenalin. Often the acid-alkaline balance plays a part here and with guidance the balance can be restored. Much can be achieved with a well-balanced diet. Patients with colitis and ulcerative colitis conditions often benefit from a wheat-free diet, sometimes preceded by a cleansing diet. With plenty of rest, fresh air and gentle breathing exercises, the situation may be reversed. Fasting is sometimes helpful and several fasting methods are described in my book *Water – Healer or Poison?*. Avoid heavily spiced foods.

The régime of Dr Vogel's liver diet seems to be well suited to colitis problems. Specific items to avoid include tap water, salt, sugar, spices, alcohol, any pork products, citrus fruits and nicotine. Recommended for colitis and ulcerative colitis patients are cooked vegetables, cooked or stewed fruits, and perhaps a salad, but this must be chewed very thoroughly. Brief dietary outlines are as follows:

Recommended foods
Raw vegetables, salads mixed with Molkosan, buttermilk, low fat yoghurt, toasted wholemeal bread, potatoes, Ryvita, sunflower or olive oil, and honey; herb tea, apple juice, beetroot juice, blackcurrant juice; natural brown rice, grapefruit, grapes and berries.

Forbidden foods
Coffee, tea, white sugar and flour (and products made with them), vinegar, tinned products, fruit other than that mentioned above, meat, fish, butter, fried food, spices, cucumber, cabbage, cauliflower and spinach; no sweets or chocolate.

Special recommendations
- Take two plates of grated carrot daily
- Walk in the fresh air for one to one and a half hours a day
- One day a week should be a fasting day; apple juice, chamomile tea or carrot juice is allowed
- Spend fifteen minutes on breathing exercises twice a day
- Always eat and drink slowly – take your time
- Avoid very hot or very cold food and drink

Recommended preparation method for whole brown rice
Put rice in a casserole or pyrex dish. Cover the rice with boiling milk or water and have the oven preheated to its highest temperature. Cook for only ten to fifteen minutes and switch off the oven. Keep rice in oven for five to six hours. Cut up some vegetables such as parsley, chicory, celery and cress and mix these through the rice with a little garlic salt. Heat it up and the rice will be ready to serve.

Rice is one of the most valuable components of this diet. These relatively simple guidelines will help to counteract the colitis problem, thus avoiding further deterioration and development of ulcerative colitis.

Colitis can occur at any stage, but it seems to mostly affect young adults of either sex. It is important that this condition should be controlled as early as possible. Fortunately, naturopathic medicine can be of great help to this condition. If the patient is aware of nutritional aspects, the body's own defence mechanism will be allowed to get on with the job.

In general it is advisable that colitis and ulcerative colitis patients seek guidance and that the condition is monitored. Further deterioration will take place if the condition goes unchecked.

It is an interesting thought that during the Second World War, in my native country the Netherlands, there were no cases of colitis or diverticulitis. This confirms the theory that diet is so important. Wheat was very difficult to obtain and gluten was eaten only in very small amounts. I always suggest a gluten-free diet for multiple sclerosis patients, and I have noticed that if they were also suffering from colitis or diverticulitis, this condition very often completely disappeared by following this diet.

It is not just multiple sclerosis patients to whom I recommend cutting out gluten. Professor Roger McDougall devised a basic diet in which white sugar, refined foods and dairy produce are avoided, as well as being completely gluten-free. Wheat is replaced by corn or rice. Indeed, I must stress that it is wheat especially that seems to be the substance that irritates colitis or ulcerative colitis patients. The gluten-free diet is explained in great detail in my book *Multiple Sclerosis*.

I must add that colitis and ulcerative colitis patients should take supplementary vitamins and here again I can wholeheartedly recommend Health Insurance Plus, the formula mentioned earlier. Gastronol and Centaurium, both Dr Vogel remedies, should also be considered.

As ulcerative colitis occurs in about 25 per cent of women during the first three months of pregnancy, guidance is definitely necessary. People with long-term ulcerative colitis must be very careful, because the deep growth of ulceration in the bowel wall may cause leakage of the colon's contents into the abdominal cavity. This can cause severe problems, while widespread ulcerative colitis will increase the risk of cancer of the colon or rectum. It could also cause extensive bleeding from tiny ulcerations. Cancer in its early stages can surreptitiously affect the membrane of the colon rectal tissue through to the mucosa and sub-mucosa. A tumour is capable of penetrating the wall of the intestines to lymph nodes or to more important organs such as the liver. This sort of cancer quite often runs in families and one should be on the alert for this.

I must also give a word of warning to people who, through bad eating habits, make the colon lazy. Constipation is usually the first alarm signal and strong drugs for constipation could easily aggravate a colitis condition. Foods with a high percentage of natural roughage, such as wholemeal bread, wholefoods and vegetables, will never cause colitis or aggravate an existing condition. Often it is the wrong kind of food that has triggered the problem. The more roughage in our food, the better the colon will be able to do its work and the better our health will be.

Constipated patients on long-term drug treatments are more likely to experience colitis problems, and it is even worse if that condition is allowed to develop into ulcerative colitis. Bowel cleansing is very important and therefore fasting and dieting are necessary for a colitis patient to improve. There should be no need for enemas or extensive colonic irrigation. Be sensible and start with revising the existing dietary régime; by doing so, the bowel is given a chance to do the job for which it was designed. If this is ignored the toxic waste that should have been eliminated may penetrate or seep through the bowel lining, the mucous membrane, back into the system. This would make things worse than ever. Again I stress that a period of fasting, even for one day a week, is very helpful. Feel free to drink fruit juices, though avoid citrus ones. Drink fruit or vegetable juices at breakfast, lunch, dinner and supper time. During the fast an enema, a hot Epsom salts bath or a mustard bath may be a good idea.

It is important that the dietary advice from the previous chapter be applied. In particular, meat, spices, alcohol, and citrus fruit should be avoided by patients who have colitis tendencies. Our food should always be chewed well, especially fruit and nuts, as in this way the colon can better tolerate the food, even if it is in an inflamed condition.

With such a delicate condition we must be selective in our choice of food and therefore organically grown produce is preferred. Wheat should be avoided, because it is quite possible that a colitis condition could develop from an irritable bowel; this can be rectified at an early stage with a wheat-free or a gluten-free diet. Please do not think that such a diet will be too restrictive. Try it first without prejudice. If you look at a cook-book for wheat-free diets, you may be pleasantly surprised. There are plenty of recipes suitable for colitis patients.

Sometimes an answer to this condition can be quite easily found. When I recently examined one of my patients I discovered that she was extremely deficient in magnesium. Although this mineral is present in natural foods, a lot of magnesium in the soil has been lost, and this is where most of our food is grown. Even more minerals are lost during the refining or processing of food. Lack of magnesium can manifest itself in chronic diarrhoea, but also in colitis or other bowel diseases. Much magnesium leaves the body in the urine and I was not terribly surprised when tests showed that this patient clearly had a magnesium deficiency. It was amazing to see how quickly her condition improved with supplementary magnesium. She readily admitted that she was a 'fast food junkie' (these were her own words), and was greatly bothered with wind problems, abdominal pains and bouts of diarrhoea. Because she had ignored the alarm signals, the result was considerable bowel inflammation and irritation.

It amazes me how often doctors still advise colitis patients to follow a milk diet, and I am in no doubt that some of these patients have aggravated their problems by following such a diet. Milk is actually quite often the instigator of their problems, especially in cases of allergic reactions.

Use olive oil in cooking because this helps the digestion, and instead of vinegar use Molkosan together with olive oil for salad dressings. This makes a tasty and healthy alternative.

In summing up, I would suggest that you experiment with some culinary herbs in your cooking, such as cumin, fennel, aniseed, thyme, sage and rosemary. Extra acidophilus will help, as will garlic, unless flatulence is a problem. B vitamins are helpful for the nervous system, just as vitamin C improves absorption. Minerals such as iron, magnesium, potassium and zinc are greatly needed. Eat soya, brown rice, millet, sesame seeds, sprouted seeds, and so on. Lastly, try out some of the fasting programmes and water treatments recommended.

Chapter 11

Diverticulitis and Diverticulosis

Unfortunately in this day and age we are seeing more and more cases of diverticulitis or diverticulosis. Diverticula are the mucosal sacculations which protrude from the intestinal lumen to the bowel wall, and are commonly found in the colon, particularly the sigmoid. If there are no complications the disorder is often described as diverticulosis, but when there is inflammation it is referred to as diverticulitis.

Diverticulosis is a weakening of the bowel wall penetrated by blood vessels. The fully developed diverticula have spherical pouches which are connected to the intestinal lumen by narrow necks. Problems here can be the result of an irritable colon or increased colonic pressure. Trouble with the sigmoid colon can be caused by pressure and toxic waste collecting in the area. The situation will greatly deteriorate if this toxicity develops into an inflammation.

Imagine the sigmoid as a little bend in the colon. (It is best visualised as the drainpipe under a sink. We know that the U-bend in the drain has to be undone from time to time in order to clear the rubbish away. I have often told patients that I wish we could undo the sigmoid U-bend occasionally to cleanse the colon of all the waste matter that has gathered there.) Food remnants trapped here cause toxicity and that can lead to grave problems. It is possible to keep the colon and the bowels clear by dietary measures. When residue or plaque has been allowed to settle, however, it is very difficult to remove. Yet, it must be done and we will feel so much better after it has been removed. An irritable colon is like an alarm and if the stools are not well-formed motions, this is yet another distress signal. Often a sigmoidoscopy will show what is happening in that part of the abdomen. It will indicate that our diet is incorrect. Here lies the cause of diverticulosis problems.

During certain stages in life we can experience digestion and absorption problems when the body needs help from digestive enzymes, nutrients, vitamins and minerals. For our general health it is of vital importance to keep that process going. It is no wonder that throughout the world there are so many gastrointestinal problems resulting in diverticulosis, since the diverticula pockets that have become established will be there to stay for life unless we do something about it.

Some doctors believe that irritable bowel syndrome is associated with diverticulosis. As I have explained, the diverticulum is a pocket and diverticulosis is a condition whereby dozens of small pockets balloon out at weak points in the wall of the colon. Diverticula mostly occur in the sigmoid colon and as this is the narrowest part it can also spread to the nearby transverse colon. It is now widely accepted that dietary management is of great influence, as this problem is so much greater in the West than in any other part of the world. Fibre must be increased in the diet and flatulence and bloated feelings should be avoided. When these problems occur patients can benefit from taking Arabiaforce, a herb preparation for stimulating stomach activity, for the promotion of appetite and for general strengthening. It is recommended for the treatment of dyspepsia, sub-acidic gastritis, stomach cramps, nausea, changes in diet and climate, and it also acts as a biliary flow stimulant.

The worst thing for either diverticulitis or diverticulosis is taking antibiotics. These should only be taken if absolutely necessary, as I have seen many problems like this created or aggravated by the use of antibiotics. Friendly bacteria in the bowels are destroyed and the condition could easily go from bad to worse.

If there is bleeding in a diverticulitis case, or even perforation, antibiotics are prescribed and the bacterial balance is upset. The diverticula become inflamed and infected, or develop into abscesses or boils. The raised pressure in the colon can cause a chronically inflamed bowel and may even lead to urinary tract infections.

Diverticulitis has been described as a left-sided appendicitis, and pain, swelling, nausea, vomiting and fever are possible symptoms. Prevention is better than cure and therefore it should be stressed that action at the very start of a diverticulosis condition is essential to prevent it developing into a much more serious problem, such as full-blown diverticulitis. Patients can alter their diet as necessary or take the correct remedies already mentioned, and gradually introduce garlic into the diet. Garlic is a wonderful food with tremendous antiseptic properties and throughout many centuries it has been eaten for its beneficial characteristics. With its powerful cleansing effects it is a formidable form of medicine. Consequently, garlic has been subjected to intensive scientific research over many years and there are many publications expounding its value for anti-bacterial, anti-tumour, anti-fungal, anti-carcinogenic, anti-arteriosclerotic action. Even for uncontrollable blood pressure variations, garlic seems to have a stabilising effect.

I remember my last visit to Dr Vogel in Switzerland, who was then already over ninety years of age. During a walk around the herb garden we saw wild garlic. Dr Vogel dug his fingers into the ground to find the bulb and cleared the soil away from it. He pointed to the silver-white bulb that had been hidden in the ground, and it was almost without blemishes or wrinkles. I discuss the specific values of garlic in my book *Traditional Home and Herbal Remedies*, and in cases of diverticulitis or diverticulosis it is of great benefit.

Chapter 12

Crohn's Disease

A patient, who is now a fellow practitioner, came to see me a number of years ago. She had been diagnosed as suffering from Crohn's disease and when I checked her family history I realised that quite a few family members had suffered tuberculosis. This was reason enough for me to prescribe the homoeopathic preparation Tuberculinum as a constitutional remedy; the response was almost unbelievable. Not unexpectedly, her condition worsened initially and then improved rapidly. When she went back to the hospital she had to explain that this tiny tablet of Tuberculinum had reversed her condition and had done such a wonderful job. It is of course up to the practitioner to select the appropriate remedy and if this choice has been correct, the remedy will be effective.

Crohn's disease is a condition of a non-specific, chronic inflammatory disease which usually affects the lower ileum, but may involve other parts of the intestines. Generally it seems to affect the younger generation, although it appears to be more common among males than females. People with full-blown Crohn's disease can suffer dreadfully, especially if the acute inflammatory process is located in the ileocaecal region. A frequently experienced symptom is diarrhoea, and in chronic Crohn's disease diarrhoea will be accompanied by severe cramps. The nature of this disease usually affects the patient emotionally and he or she may become very insecure.

When the illness is in an active phase one of its most distressing symptoms is lack of bowel control. This is why the National Association for Colitis and Crohn's Disease has produced a

'Can't Wait' card, which is available to all sufferers and explains why the card-carrier must have immediate access to a toilet.

Apart from the distress and humiliation caused by attacks of diarrhoea, patients often lose weight due to poor appetite, and anaemia can result if blood is lost regularly. In order to make a diagnosis a specialist will need to take a direct look at the lining of the ileum. These tests may be undergone at an out-patient clinic and include various methods:

- A sigmoidoscopy, when a short, illuminated tube or flexible telescope is passed into the colon via the anus so that the doctor may see the colon and rectum. Tiny samples of tissue may be taken for analysis at the same time.
- A colonoscopy, which is an examination of the whole colon using a fibre-optic viewing instrument passed through the anus.
- A barium enema, where barium liquid is run into the bowel through the anus and X-rays are taken.
- A barium follow-through, when barium liquid is swallowed and X-ray pictures are taken of the small intestine.

Diagnosis will decide the treatment. Acute conditions may subside spontaneously. However, if a chronic condition has been diagnosed, progress will be slow. Again diet is very important, as are vitamins, minerals and trace elements. As with many similar problems, Crohn's disease is also called regional enteritis. I have seen encouraging results with the remedies Centaurium, Tormentavena and Petasan.

It was with great pleasure that I encouraged my former patient to train to become a practitioner. She claimed that she was so delighted with her remarkable recovery, thanks to a simple constitutional remedy, that she had become obsessed with the idea of practising medicine.

As with other abdominal problems, the diet for a Crohn's disease patient must be rich in fibre. Poor digestion can contribute to the problem. Changes in the diet or lifestyle may result in a temporary remission. For example, it is quite usual for a Crohn's disease sufferer to experience no symptoms throughout her pregnancy, but after the baby is born the symptoms may recur severely.

In the case of an inflammatory bowel disease that has been diagnosed as either colitis or Crohn's disease, inflammation may affect the mouth, oesophagus, stomach, duodenum, appendix and anus. It is therefore very worrying to know that it can continue for the rest of one's life if nothing is done about it.

It is my belief that Crohn's disease is often caused by miasmas left from previous inflammations, viruses or infections. This was also the case with the patient I mentioned at the beginning of this chapter where the miasma was caused by the hereditary tuberculosis.

Often with Crohn's disease patients, we find that there is an allergy to milk and dairy products. These should be immediately prohibited from the diet upon diagnosis, and all Crohn's disease patients must be careful with highly spiced foods, alcohol, nicotine, and sometimes citrus fruits. Gentle exercise, rest and relaxation are necessary and for this purpose Hara breathing exercises (which are described in great detail in my book *Stress and Nervous Disorders*) are especially valuable. Stress can cause a dark red or black colour through the presence of blood in the stool. The small intestine may be bleeding and this is certainly the time to take action and contact one's doctor. The condition must be correctly diagnosed because ulcerative colitis symptoms are quite similar to Crohn's disease. Although colitis only affects the colon, Crohn's disease will affect any part or even the whole of the digestive canal, and therefore treatment must be different.

There are various schools of thought on both problems. Investigations have concluded that the problems can be caused by bacteria or a virus, or possibly a weakness in the immune system. The condition often develops between the ages of fifteen and forty, but I have also seen babies and very young children who had such problems. To reach the correct diagnosis some of the recently developed investigative equipment and methods are very helpful. Allow me to stress how important it is to explore the treatment options and recommendations if you are diagnosed as suffering from this disease.

Natural treatment is not only more gentle, but is also extremely effective. I would recommend that the supplement Imuno-Strength be taken in combination with good dietary management. This is a remedy from Nature's Best designed to boost the immune system so that it is able to deal with viruses, bacteria and toxins before they become established. Today's world is full of challenges to our defence mechanism. Some of these challenges – such as the food we eat, the stresses and strains of work – are under our control, others are not. These include environmental pollution by potentially toxic chemicals. In these circumstances it makes sense to help protect the integrity of our immune system by safeguarding our nutrition. As well as carefully selected amounts of the vitamins and minerals known to be needed for the effective functioning of the immune system, Imuno-Strength contains the very special herbs Devil's Claw and Echinacea, which I prescribe in various different combinations. Imuno-Strength contains:

Vitamin A	900mcg
Riboflavin (vitamin B$_2$)	10mg
Vitamin B$_6$	50mg
Folic acid	50mcg
Pantothenic acid	50mg
Vitamin C	165mg
Vitamin E	80 iu
Calcium	19mg
Iron	1mg
Magnesium	3mg
Manganese	500mcg
Selenium	100mcg
Zinc	15mg
Devil's Claw	100mg
Echinacea purpurea	200mg
Siberian Ginseng	15mg

I often prescribe supplementary vitamin B$_{12}$ if I consider this necessary for the patient. Herbal teas are good, and chamomile tea in particular helps this condition. For generations this tea has been used for anti-inflammatory purposes and it is helpful for stomach ailments as well as for fevers and colds. After scientific investigations during recent decades chamomile has become known for its anti-peptic, anti-spasmodic, anti-bacterial and anti-fungal characteristics, which makes it quite special. It is not just a herb with some curative properties, but it also makes a very nice drink. It can really help sufferers of Crohn's disease, and with the correct remedies much can be done to make life easier.

Chapter 13

Coeliac Disease

Not so long ago I said goodbye for the last time to one of my best friends. I felt her loss deeply, because she was a dear friend and a very interesting lady. Moreover, I felt that her death was unnecessary. This patient was a mystery to orthodox practitioners, as she was for me too. She had had so many medical tests that it sometimes surprised me that she could still be bothered. Somehow she never displayed the typical symptoms of coeliac disease. She certainly seemed to do reasonably well under my treatment, but the time came when I also had to ask her to take further tests. As time passed, I was mystified by her illness and although she felt slightly better than she had, I was convinced that something was seriously wrong.

I am sure that the symptoms of this extremely unpleasant illness have mystified many doctors, and although in some forms it is relatively easy to diagnose, with this lady it remained a mystery until the very end. Unfortunately, after her liver had been permanently damaged, she suddenly remembered that when she was younger she had suffered from coeliac disease. By then, unfortunately, it was too late and she never reached middle age.

I was upset that no proper diagnosis was reached and it continues to puzzle me that coeliac disease can remain undiagnosed. Coeliac disease is damage to the intestinal lining and subsequent impairment of the digestion. It is characterised by the inability to digest cereals containing gluten, that is wheat, rye, barley and oats, as well as by poor absorption of other nutrients. The disease can sometimes be traced back to being given cereal as a baby before the intestines are developed. Unfortunately, the condition is permanent and can recur at any time in life as an allergy to cereals. My friend was a pleasant and mild-natured person, who always looked a little too pale. As I said, she suddenly remembered that as a child she had suffered from digestive problems, although for many years no clear symptoms had been apparent. With hindsight it was possibly because of the trauma of losing her son in a road accident that her old allergy to gluten recurred. An established allergy nearly always remains with the person concerned, but allergies can often be controlled if the immune system is strong. Trauma, however, can upset this situation.

A similar problem happened with another good friend, but he was fortunately diagnosed quickly, because he clearly remembered his previous allergy problems. As a child he had had quite a few allergic reactions, but he thought he had outgrown them. That is until he went through a very stressful stage in his life with his business, and a few traumatic experiences brought the whole thing back again. We now understand that this is often a problem with coeliac disease: it is not always correctly diagnosed and thus remains unrecognised, with the result that it is not treated correctly. However, when diagnosed, vitamin B-complex is often recommended as a supplement. As happened to both my friends, patients usually lose weight and their stools become bulky and pale, alternating from constipation to diarrhoea. By then, the signs of nutritional deficiencies are clear. Again digestion and absorption are at the root of the problem.

Most medical books claim that an uncomplicated case of coeliac disease is rarely fatal, yet my dear friend proved this to be wrong. Coeliac disease, also unheard of during the Second World War in the Netherlands, is now very much on the increase and I consider wheat protein as the main enemy. Hyperactivity was identified in experiments with rats by Dr E. W. Williams of the University College of North Wales. In these tests it was demonstrated that the intestinal villi of rats whose diet included wheat protein changed from being long and slender into a shorter, more squat shape. With this knowledge it can be seen that rice is a much better nutrient than wheat for a coeliac patient. I would even go so far as to suggest that this is the case for everyone. The gluten-free diet which I worked out with Prof Roger McDougall is most suitable for a coeliac person. Like multiple sclerosis patients, the coeliac patient must be careful not to lose too much weight: they should eat plenty of potatoes, bananas, nuts and the kind of food that will keep the weight steady and balanced. Although like everyone else many coeliac patients have a fondness for cereals, I must stress that these are dangerous for them.

Why is gluten intolerance found in so many people? Gluten is a generic term for two proteins, prolamine and glutain, which are found in different grains. A gluten intolerance is usually caused by wheat, rye, oats, barley or buckwheat, and manifests itself primarily as an allergy or an irritation in the small intestine. This is possibly due to a deficiency of enzymes, vitamins, minerals or even trace elements. A gluten intolerance can cause many things, from diarrhoea to a loss of appetite, or to coeliac disease. Coeliac patients can sometimes tolerate certain grains, but they definitely cannot cope with wheat. So it is important for the coeliac patient to follow fairly strict dietary rules.

A more detailed description of the gluten-free diet can be found in my book *Multiple Sclerosis* and I will therefore not repeat too much of it here. It is sufficient to state my belief that the dietary approach to degenerative conditions should take the form of a four-pronged attack:

- No gluten
- Low sugars
- Low animal fats and high unsaturated fats
- Supplementing possible vitamin and mineral deficiencies.

It is medically accepted that certain conditions are caused or aggravated by the consumption of certain foods. For example, coeliac disease is linked with cereals, diabetes and hypoglycaemia with sugar, and cardio-vascular conditions with dairy fats. I believe that by eating the correct food patients have a good chance of improving their condition. Success depends on your own determination, and when the decision has been made to follow the rules, half-hearted measures are not enough. Once you have decided to change your diet, adhere to the instructions or else the effort will not be worth while. Remember that diet is only a matter of habit and that at all times the choice is yours.

I have seen coeliac patients gain long-term remission, after which the symptoms suddenly flare up again for no apparent reason. However, it is possible to control this quickly, once the offending factor has been removed. Apart from diet, there are also several natural remedies to help the coeliac patient, namely Pancreatin from Nature's Best and Tormentavena and Echinaforce from Bioforce.

Coeliac sufferers are also advised to eat natural yoghurt which should always agree with them and improve their condition. Understandably, the patient may get bored sometimes with the fairly strict dietary guidelines, but remember that a coeliac patient need not suffer: as long as the rules are obeyed, the reward will be increased energy and better health. At such times I quote Calvin Coolidge to coeliac patients: 'Persistence and determination are omnipotent'.

Chapter 14

Constipation

A fifty-two-year-old patient explained to me that for some time he had experienced problems with constipation, although he used to have most regular bowel movement. He had sought my help because he still felt the urge to move his bowels and yet was unable to do so. This gentleman probably would have carried on without seeking help if he hadn't noticed some blood in his stools a few days previously. He was worried that he might be suffering from internal haemorrhoids and therefore he made an appointment to see me. I only wish that I could have diagnosed haemorrhoids, because in fact his medical condition was far more serious. The alternating constipation, the occasional loose stools and the blood loss indicated cancer. I told him that he required specialist help and fortunately his general practitioner immediately referred him to hospital, where a malignant tumour was diagnosed and he had surgery.

The occurrence of bowel cancer in Scotland is statistically frightening, and the lives of thousands of people are claimed by it every year. In most cases the large intestine is affected and very often by the time this disease has been diagnosed, the condition is too far advanced for the surgeon to be able to operate successfully. More can be read about these conditions in my book *Cancer and Leukaemia*, but it should be clear to the reader that if blood is passed with a bowel movement, a physician must be consulted immediately. Fortunately, nowadays surgery is very advanced and quite often the tumour can be removed successfully if timely action is taken. Control over the bowel movement may be restored, although this is not always the case and should not be taken for granted. If the only option is to remove the anus, a colostomy becomes necessary. Of course a metastasis may be discovered which will complicate matters, but otherwise the patient's lifestyle can be adapted to suit the change in circumtances.

Cancer of the large intestine is usually discovered because of pain in the stomach, motions alternating between hard stools and diarrhoea, and blood in the stools. These signs should not be ignored, because if a serious condition is developing, it should be attended to as early as possible.

The reason I mentioned the gentleman with constipation problems is because this is a typical example of early symptoms. Very often cancerous conditions originate in the bowel and it is part of the elimination process, mentioned in the first chapter, which must function correctly. There is no need for the digestive system to function incorrectly if only we take action to regulate this process. What is imported must be exported within twenty-four hours or else we are constipated. A bowel movement should take place daily and if this is not the case remedial action must be taken. Usually the absence of a daily motion is due to dietary mismanagement, or a lifestyle in which the bowels are unable to cope.

I remember when Dr Vogel and I opened our first naturopathic clinic. On the top floor of the clinic a monstrous piece of equipment was installed for the purpose of bowel cleansing. At any one of those treatment sessions about sixty pints of chamomile water were passed through the bowels of the patient. I always made sure that the patient saw what was removed, because very few people realise how much matter is retained in the bowels. The reader may now understand why impaired bowel functions can lead to diverse medical conditions such as Candida albicans, Crohn's disease and ulcers.

It always amazed me to hear how well people felt after a bowel cleansing session. Some patients actually asked eagerly when the next treatment session would be allowed. This, however, is part of the problem, because the bowels should perform this function spontaneously rather than depending on external aid. Certain conditions most certainly benefit from higher bowel cleansing treatment, while colonic irrigation may also be beneficial. However, if we behave in a responsible way with our diet, it is unlikely that these cleansing processes should be required, because the body takes care of this in its own way. Many problems nowadays occur because the balance of friendly bacteria and mucus in the bowel is disturbed. Sometimes such a disturbance can be easily overcome by a food supplement such as Dr Vogel's Linoforce. The linseeds, coated with herbal substances, result in a regular gentle bowel movement and will regenerate the bowels by reintroducing mucus into this function. Recently, during a lecture tour in Australia, I placed one of these seeds on my hand and blew it away. I told the audience that I would give some of them a single seed to chew and they would experience how the mucus production was stimulated. Linoforce needs to be taken twice a day and I maintain that this is one of the finest remedies to restore good bowel management.

Enemas are beneficial, especially a coffee enema (the exact instructions can be found in my book *Cancer and Leukaemia*). I remember listening to a lecture by Dr Max Gerson who stated categorically that he thought coffee performed a better service to one's health if it was used at the other end of the body – that is, instead of drinking coffee, it would be much more advantageous healthwise if it were used as an enema, because it cleanses the bowels so well.

So, what do we do if we have constipation? On my last visit to Canada I discussed this topic at length with one of my best friends, whom I regard as one of the leading authorities on the subject of colonic irrigation. She suggested that I should attend a colonic irrigation session and I saw the mass of material that was removed from the body, but I was somewhat concerned about the mucus that was also removed from the bowel. She agreed, and told me that after colonic irrigation people are advised to take acidophilus. This is essential because the gastrointestinal tract of a normal healthy individual plays host to a very large and varied population of micro-organisms. In an adult the total weight of bacteria will amount to approximately one kilogramme. The distribution and type of bacteria varies considerably throughout the intestine. At the top end – the stomach and small intestine – bacteria numbers are relatively low due to the high acidity of the stomach which kills most of the bacteria we ingest with our food. However, at the other end of the gastrointestinal tract, especially in the colon, there is a massive concentration of bacteria. In healthy individuals this microbial population is delicately balanced and the gastrointestinal tract can only function effectively if this balance is maintained.

The quality of the body's intestinal flora is determined by the balance between the various microbial species, especially the two predominant groups, the Bifido bacteria and the Bacteroides bacteria. Bifido species are regarded as beneficial and tend to counterbalance the putrefactive Bacteroides bacteria. The bacteria balance should remain stable throughout life, although certain factors – such as illness, excessive yeast growth, dietary changes, travelling abroad or treatments with antibiotics – can upset the balance. It has also been shown that in the elderly, Bifido bacteria often decreases significantly, which may account for age-related changes in the working of the gastrointestinal tract.

The principle of supporting the beneficial bacteria with supplements containing viable bacteria was established in the 1970s. Since then the supplements have become more and more sophisticated and Nature's Best now offers probably the most up-to-date version available in the UK. Nature's Best Acidophilus Plus consists of human-strain *Lactobacillus acidophilus* and *Lactobacillus bifudus*. Each capsule contains one billion biologically active micro-organisms; it is dairy-free and particularly popular with those on yeast-free diets. The gelatine capsules can be opened easily and the powder contents sprinkled on food by those wishing to avoid animal products altogether.

My friend, the colonic specialist, especially recommends colonic irrigation for the elderly, and with her kind permission I quote some details from her clinic's brochure:

> The colon irrigation is a procedure carried out to irrigate the lower bowel with water to remove faeces, mucus and toxic material. It is done as a procedure with direct benefits to the colon and digestive system and as a concomitant procedure to other treatments, such as chiropractice, naturopathy, massage and gastroenterology, in order to make them easier or more effective.

Equipment

A proctosyringe or similarly named irrigation device consists of a stainless steel cylinder (pipe) with one end shaped as a truncated cone and the other straight. An obturator fits through the cylinder to allow easy entry of the instrument through the anus into the rectum. A smaller cylinder is attached on the side to allow entry of water and a flange is placed around the large cylinder closer to the cone end to limit entry. Rubber tubing for water supply and waste and a container for a gravity-fed water source complete the essential equipment. All equipment should be capable of sterilisation or be disposable.

Introduction of water

Water flows continuously through the instrument and is introduced into the colon by blocking the waste tube. A method of counting is used to determine the distance the water has travelled in the colon. The colon condition is assessed by the irrigationist who will determine the distance the water will reach in a given time. Determination of the time needed to release the waste tube is based on a schedule of increasing water into the colon, but is always overridden by the client's indication that pressure tolerance is reached. Standards include selecting correct water temperature based on evaluation of the colon, determining when to release the water, and so on.

Massage

This is a highly important aspect of colonic irrigation and is more difficult to learn, just as any examination of the abdomen is one of the most difficult techniques to learn. The colon irrigationist must know the various organs by touch and be able to tell to some degree the status of the colon, for example, location, size, shape, contents (gases, liquids, solids) and activity. The aim of the massage is to facilitate the removal of matter from the colon by the water and is even more important in those cases which are most difficult due to atonicity, spasticity, disease, and so on. Standards include applying the minimum massage to gain the desired effect, being able to identify the organs in the abdomen, especially the digestive system and identifying the status of the colon.

Treatment

A typical treatment requires the constant attention of the colon irrigationist. Leaving a client attached to a colon irrigation machine for a half-hour without being in attendance is not recommended. The course of a treatment normally concludes by bringing water around to the caecum and flushing it out. With care and attention this can be done in about forty-five minutes. Whether the flushing of the caecum occurs or not, the client should in no case be treated longer than an hour, since after that length of time the client can become exhausted. An important aspect of the treatment is being able to interpret the usual condition and current state of the colon by observation of the effluent from the colon during the treatment. This is observed through a tubular 'window' which is part of the waste tubing. Observation and interpretation allow ongoing modification of the treatment procedure. Standards for the treatment include adapting the treatment to the individual case so that co-operation is evident from the client and no adverse effects are reported to the therapist which are not ameliorated.

Sterile procedure

Sterilisation of instruments and equipment is crucial to proper procedure and also instils confidence in the client. Mechanical cleaning of instruments should be complete and they should be subsequently chemically or heat sterilised. A good quality of surgical stainless steel is recommended for instruments. The standard for the instruments is that no bacteria can be cultured from them.

Effectiveness

The therapy is invasive only in the strict medical sense that an instrument physically enters the body. It is not chemically or procedurally invasive and it is certainly not an aggressive therapy if done correctly. The therapy produces a gradual restoration of the colon to full function and so its effectiveness cannot usually be measured over a short period of time. The standard for the effectiveness of an individual treatment might include the material that was removed from the colon, the client reported no discomfort as a result of the colonic irrigation, and the client also reported feeling positive effects from the colonic treatment. The standard for effectiveness for a longer series of colonic treatments would include reporting better elimination, improved overall health, and relief from specific ailments which were not undergoing any other treatment.

Earlier, I indicated that colonic irrigation is advisable especially for the elderly. This is because they seem to be more prone to constipation, most likely because they are physically less active. However, we should not overlook the fact that very often babies and toddlers up to the age of four are also prone to constipation. Individuals have different expectations. As a rule, we should have a bowel movement every day, although I know that for quite a few people a bowel movement every second day is quite acceptable. Whatever the established pattern, it should be understood that any change from a previously existing routine is noteworthy, because this may be an indication of changes in the body.

A forty-year-old female patient came to see me about weight problems. Her weight hovered around the 18-stone mark and it was obvious that she was uncomfortable. Her lips were slightly blue and upon checking I was not surprised to see that her blood pressure was 220/140. Furthermore, I also diagnosed clear evidence of tachycardia. What does a practitioner do in such a case, apart from hoping that the patient will not collapse in his consulting rooms or clinic? Immediate action was required. I asked her when she last had a bowel movement. She was insistent that she was not constipated, because she went to the toilet two or three times a week. Eventually I managed to convince my patient that this was not sufficient and that she required a good bowel cleansing programme and a sensible diet. Within a surprisingly short time her blood pressure normalised.

In an article published by Bioforce, constipation is explained as a situation where the large intestine retains food remnants, thus allowing toxins which would normally pass through the body within twenty-four hours to be absorbed. This causes an accumulation of toxins in the body, over-burdening the liver. The result can be tiredness, listlessness, skin impurities and increased susceptibility to illness. The intestines, pancreas and liver suffer from blockages because insufficient matter is eliminated from the body. Please note that cellulose, a substance present in grains and vegetables, acts like a brush moving through the intestines, and if the patient is constipated this function cannot be performed.

The following are among the possible causes of constipation:

- dietary errors and lack of fibre
- insufficient physical exercise
- poor respiration
- physical causes
- specific medication
- poor stomach and intestinal function
- liver and gall bladder dysfunction
- hormonal disruption

The reader must understand that during pregnancy, the taking of laxatives is unwise. Most laxatives work on the basis that the intestinal area is sufficiently irritated to encourage the body to eliminate waste matter. However, this irritation can also encompass the womb. Only laxative remedies which act as a gentle softener may be used during pregnancy, and even then only after consultation with one's general practitioner. General therapeutic advice is:

- keep to a suitable time every day to attempt to pass a motion and allow sufficient time
- take more physical exercise
- do not use the same laxatives for months on end
- avoid food that lacks fibre and products that contain white sugar
- eat raw vegetables (especially cabbage varieties), plums, prunes, grapes, raspberries, figs, cherries and strawberries
- add a teaspoon of bran to each meal
- drink two glasses of lukewarm water first thing each morning

Remedies favoured by Dr Vogel for the treatment of constipation depend upon the patient's individual circumstances and should be taken according to the advice of the practitioner. The choice from the Bioforce range of medication is plentiful, including Linoforce, Frangula, Aloe complex UA, Curcuma complex, Boldocynara, and Nux vomica D4.

I have mentioned several times already that fibre will stimulate bowel movement in a completely natural way. Fibre is a vitally important part of our diet and doctors and nutritionists agree that most people living in developed countries do not eat enough of it. Fibre is nearly always derived from plants and consists of a variety of different compounds. Nutritionists now describe fibre compounds as either soluble or insoluble, the distinction being made since each type has a different activity. Both types, however, share one important property: they are not digested (broken up by intestinal enzymes) and therefore pass into the bowel unabsorbed. During the passage through the intestines they combine with water, bile salts and impurities, the latter being produced by bacteria in the lower gut.

Soluble fibre consists of compounds such as gums, pectins and mucilages, and when they dissolve in water they form gelatinous compounds which are particularly good at binding to bile salts. These salts are produced in the liver from cholesterol and are secreted into the gut (via the gall bladder) where they assist in the digestion of fats. They are then reabsorbed further down the intestine and recycled through the liver. However, some of the bile salts become bound with dietary fibre, and therefore fail to become reabsorbed. In response to this the body has to use blood cholesterol to replace the 'lost' bile salts. It is in this way that soluble fibre, and to a lesser extent insoluble fibre, play their part in removing cholesterol from the body. Insoluble fibre is usually cellulose and has a bulking action, helping to speed the passage of food through the intestine and bowel.

When the importance of fibre was first realised, attention focused on bran (the husks of cereals) since it was the activity of insoluble fibre that was first acclaimed. However, nutritionists now understand the importance of soluble fibre and sources such as sugarbeet, psyllium and guar have been extensively investigated. As a result of the outcome of these investigations Nature's Best have launched a product called Toasted Fibre Flakes, made entirely from sugarbeet fibres. Its composition compared with bran is shown below:

97

	Wheat Bran	*Toasted Fibre Flakes*
Soluble fibre	3.2%	32.2%
Insoluble fibre	38.4%	48.1%
Total fibre	41.6%	80.3%

It is apparent from these figures that not only are Toasted Fibre Flakes ten times higher in soluble fibre than bran, but significantly higher in insoluble fibre as well.

The average diet contains 20 grammes of fibre daily, whereas the Department of Health recommends 30 grammes. Therefore, something in the region of 10 grammes a day of Toasted Fibre Flakes will make a very real contribution to the daily intake of soluble and insoluble fibre. The golden brown flakes resemble breadcrumbs and can be used in baking for crumble tops, biscuits and bread-making or mixed in soups, stews and casseroles. An even easier way is to sprinkle the flakes on breakfast cereals where a dessertspoonful (approximately 5 grammes) can be taken without affecting the meal.

I hope I have made it clear that constipation can be caused by many factors. It may be something we have contracted from food or long-term drugs, sedatives or tranquillisers. Even inhaled toxic matter can result in constipation. This part of our body chemistry requires care and we must take note of changes in the pattern of bowel movements. Occasionally extra help may be required and in these cases I prescribe Colon Care Plus, a supplement for colon health, to some of my patients. Nature's Best Colon Care Plus is not a laxative, but a combination which includes several herbs, vegetable fibre and probiotic bacteria. This formula is designed to help a healthy colon maintain optimum levels of nutrient absorption and elimination of waste. The colon, or large intestine, is designed to expedite waste matter from the body and is also involved in the absorption of nutrients from food. For the maintenance of health depends on being kept free from stale waste (which is attracted to the many crevices of the intestine), on healthy muscle tone in the colon walls, and on the presence of the correct types and proportions of resident bacteria.

In these modern times, because of the large amount of refined, processed foods in our daily diets, an effective colon care programme is important. The traditional methods of colon cleansing such as enemas, fastings and colonic irrigation do not appeal to everyone. A responsible eating programme may require more than replenishing the missing dietary fibre. Colon Care Plus uses natural ingredients to form a friendlier health technology. It consists of fourteen specially selected ingredients combined in unique form including ten different herbs, carefully selected for their broad spectrum of activity. One of these herbs, Chapparal, a traditional North American Indian herb, is reputed to have an active ingredient that specifically helps to maintain the balance of the natural fermentation processes in the colon. As the herbs do their work, Colon Care Plus also provides Probiotic 4, a unique form of friendly *Lactobacillus acidophilus* bacteria to maintain a favourable bacterial balance.

I would also like to draw the reader's attention to the fact that people with atonic constipation, which usually occurs with aged or invalid patients, must pay special attention to their diet. One such, a patient of mine, had considerable problems with this condition but taking Linoforce three times daily after a meal helped him considerably. He also changed his diet and ate muesli for breakfast mixed with yoghurt and four prunes which had been soaked overnight.

Dealing with babies and infants who suffer constipation is sometimes more difficult. Dietary approach is again important, and sometimes small amounts of Oil of Evening Primrose can be helpful, or a castor oil pack. This is a piece of linen sprinkled with castor oil which is placed over the stomach. Although it seems unlikely, this works very well for babies and infants. Elderly people can also benefit from taking castor oil, which helps to cleanse the bowels.

Lack of exercise is another important factor in causing constipation. In order to increase or decrease peristaltic contraction to relieve diarrhoea or constipation, it is important to take a certain amount of physical exercise. Walking, swimming, deep breathing exercises, in fact anything that reduces stress will lead to the relief of constipation. This is often the case with elderly people, where because of lack of exercise these problems occur. Oil of Evening Primrose relaxes and levels out the hormonal imbalances which often contribute towards constipation. Quite often in the later months of pregnancy we see problems with constipation, which can be caused by the growing foetus pressing on the rectum and other organs. At all times during pregnancy, laxatives should only be taken on professional advice. Drink plenty of liquids. Nothing could be more simple than drinking one or two glasses of lukewarm water before breakfast, yet this can be very helpful. Adding prunes to your breakfast cereal is also beneficial.

As I have said, the chemistry in the body must be balanced. In a recent report, I again read that constipation could be linked to cancer. Dr Eileen King, researcher at the University of California School of Medicine in San Francisco, has released the results of a study she conducted recently. The study concerned 1,481 women with breast cancer, or with a high risk of developing the disease. The research group included women between the ages of twenty and seventy years. Severely constipated women had a much higher incidence of abnormal cells in their breast fluid. These are the cells that are closely associated with breast cancer. In women who had two or more bowel movements a day, only about 5 per cent had abnormal cells in the fluid. When bowel elimination dropped to every day or every other day, the incidence increased to 10 per cent. With bowel movements only twice a week, the increase in cells related to breast cancer rose to 23 per cent.

Based upon this report and other studies, it must be assumed that with chronic constipation there is an increased risk of breast cancer, according to Dr King. It has been concluded that cancer-causing agents, formed in the intestines, result from constipation and are absorbed into the bloodstream. To prevent constipation the women are advised to eat a diet high in fibre, with lots of fresh vegetables and fruits. A diet containing a lot of meat tends to be constipating. According to Dr King, a healthy diet with plenty of raw fruit and vegetables could well have an influence on whether or not a woman develops breast cancer. She added that she does not favour the use of laxatives, if it can possibly be avoided.

Holistic doctors from various disciplines have recognised that the risk not only of breast cancer but of all cancer and other degenerative disease can result from poor elimination. Putrefaction, resulting from incomplete digestion, leads to poor assimilation and incomplete elimination, directly related to 'auto-intoxication' or self-poisoning of the bloodstream. Such poisons or toxins then accumulate in the areas of lowest resistance, forming a medium for the growth of viruses, bacteria and/or parasites, with consequent hypoxia or oxygen deprivation. If the consequent degenerative condition happens to be cancer, the lump or bump is the result of a usually long period of pre-disease, or pre-cancer, while the primary condition was systemic and not removed by excising the lump, unless followed by 'detoxification' and correcting the previous malfunctions in digestion, assimilation and elimination, plus a nutritious diet.

Only the body can heal, and to quote one of my favourite sayings, 'Nothing is so uncommon as common sense'. An open mind is similar to a healthy intestine that accepts food, digests it, retains what is needed, and expels the excess. A closed mind, paralysed by orthodoxy, is similar to constipation of reason, causing stifled progress and growth.

Sometimes people become neurotic about their bowel regularity, but it is important to remember that we are all different and that there are extremely few people who are blessed with a totally regular bowel movement. Laxatives must never be abused. Be sensible if you feel you require them. If possible, try increasing the fibre content of your diet, because quite apart from being beneficial for constipation, people on a high fibre diet are four times less likely to die of heart disease. In the USA the increase in the demand for laxatives is very worrying. The underlying outcome of cause and effect has been overlooked and common sense is very important in getting to grips with constipation.

Common sense dictates that if the bowels work efficiently, it is more likely that the body will function efficiently.

Chapter 15

Food Allergies

Since I wrote *Viruses, Allergies and the Immune System* some years ago I have noted that, unfortunately, the list of common allergies has grown even further – in fact, I am appalled when I think how much that list has grown since my graduation in 1959. However, we do not need too much imagination to come up with a plausible explanation as to why this should be so. Man needs food, air and water to remain alive, and the unfortunate pollution of the last two affects the quality of our food, which is cultivated under these adverse circumstances. Food allergies are therefore more common than ever. A weakened immune system is the result of interference in the growing of our food.

How does one deal with allergies? In my Harley Street clinic I see colleagues who ask me how a naturopathic practitioner approaches allergies. My answer is always that I do not treat allergies, but that I concentrate instead on the immune system. In caring for the immune system, I first of all aim to isolate the allergy. This can be done by an elimination diet or by various kinds of allergy testing, for example blood, hair or skin tests. Over the years it has been my experience that by treating the immune system many allergies will spontaneously disappear. Please don't think for a minute that I underestimate allergies; I fully understand how careful we have to be with a wheat allergy, or any allergy for that matter. It is very unwise to ignore an allergy, as that initially harmless allergy may eventually develop into a full-blown degenerative disease. We must also get used to the idea that sometimes we may be allergic to wheat or milk, for example, while a week later they cause no adverse effects. This is because the immune system changes with every tick of the clock.

I am on very good terms with one of the finest immunologists in Great Britain and we have often discussed the matter together. Neither of us professes to understand the immune system fully: although much research has been undertaken on the subject, there remain many questions. At this point I must say that in other parts of the world where I have worked or visited, I have seen many less allergic reactions than in our own country. I think this is because of a more natural diet and a more relaxed, and therefore more healthy, lifestyle. Our 'civilised' food – in other words processed and preserved food – probably causes more damage than we would like to admit. This just goes to show that we have to be prepared to change our ideas about allergies.

The body works according to various kinds of mechanisms. For example, the nervous system and the internal secretion system need to work in total harmony as the body's defence system is dependent on this. Here is the first problem: we know that air contains many bacteria, which, when they invade the body, must be removed or rendered harmless. If we are defeated in this battle, problems will occur.

The inflammatory reaction of an allergy is a sign that the body's living defence system is overreacting. Leukocytes, our internal 'soldiers', inhabit the body from top to toe and they remain on the alert for any substances invading the body. They are very much involved in our defence system. This is why, in the case of allergies, I insist on treating the immune system: I feel that with healthy dietary management we can influence and prepare this defence system to cope with toxins or invaders. Secondly, there are natural remedies which can assist and strengthen the immune system to overcome allergies. If we take a sensible approach, there is no reason why our immune or defence system should be helpless against invaders.

With great interest I followed some tests that were undertaken in Japan at the Teikyo University. These tests were designed to prove that certain materials and herbs can adjust the body's defence system to balance inflammations and allergies.

Even though allergic reactions are definitely more common,

this is still a much maligned phrase. There are many people who casually claim to be allergic to something, and yet they happily continue in their old ways. I agree that certain invaders can indeed cause very real problems, a classic example of which is pollen, which results in hay fever. Milk also often causes allergic reactions. Wheat or gluten is likely to be an allergen for people with coeliac disease. However, with specific tests it is possible to determine which nutrient or matter disagrees, and often a well-balanced diet can help the defence system to rid the body of allergy problems. The body has its own distress signals, such as constipation or diarrhoea, pains or a bloated feeling, which immediately give an indication that there may be an allergy. The process of elimination will help to identify the offending factor. The inherent chemistry of the body will react to this allergy in the same way as healthy people react to a poison.

On the whole it is understood that in the case of an allergy, something must be eliminated from the diet or the immediate environment, but little thought is given to the possibility that an allergic reaction can also be caused by a deficiency. Whatever the cause, the results can be equally distressing and the damage can be just as severe. I must stress that in trying to support the defence system, many allergies may disappear.

People are always more likely to experience an allergic reaction when they are under stress. At the present time, with the alarming unemployment figures and the general recession, allergy problems are on the increase because of stressful situations. Sometimes an elimination diet may lead to the detection of the cause, and exclusion of the offending allergens may be enough to reverse the condition. However, because allergy symptoms can be so variable, I must emphasise that the guidance of a doctor or practitioner who has experience in this field is essential. I have to insist on this because quite often I have come across stomach and bowel problems caused by allergic reactions to previously well-tolerated nutrients, in fact perfectly acceptable foodstuffs.

I am always somewhat reluctant to recommend strict rules for a general diet, just in case of food allergies. Of immediate importance is that any specific allergen is isolated. To achieve this, a food allergy elimination diet is very important and to this end I follow with the four phases of a diet designed by Dr

McKarness, based upon his work with Action Against Allergy.

Food Allergy Elimination Diet

Phase I
For five days take only lamb, pears, Malvern water and sea salt.

Phase II
Carefully reintroduce foods as directed below. If the symptoms return or the pulse rate rises by ten beats per minute or more from the pre-recorded resting pulse rate, the food introduced can be identified as the allergen. As the allergic reaction can last up to three days, return to the diet already identified as safe for three days before proceeding to test additional foods.

Day 6   Introduce broccoli and/or lettuce
Day 7   Introduce haddock or cod and carrots
Day 8   Introduce avocado pear and/or melon
Day 9   Introduce tap water and grapefruit
Day 10   Introduce cabbage and/or celery
Day 11   Introduce beef and/or plaice
Day 12   Introduce apples and/or peaches
Day 13   Introduce green grapes and herbs or China tea (without milk or sugar)

Once a food has been established as safe, it can be eaten or left out at one's personal preference.

Phase III
Endeavour to establish a balanced diet by introducing potatoes, millet, whole rice, fresh vegetables (except tomatoes) and fresh fruit (excpet oranges) into the diet. Introduce each food separately on a daily basis, testing for an increase in the pulse rate. Subsequently reintroduce pulses and rye crispbreads in small amounts and further types of sea fish besides haddock, plaice and cod.

Phase IV
Test for small amounts of foods one would wish to eat occasionally by checking the pulse rate after eating the test food alone against the background of a well-established diet.

There are all kinds of ways in which we can discover where the allergy problem lies. Last week I met a patient who was very happy after it was finally established that she was allergic to honey. The source of her problem had eluded us for some time, because honey is generally a most acceptable food, but this person was extremely allergic to honey and suffered severe stomach pains and feelings of nausea whenever she ate it. Despite the fact that she was very fond of this food, she was delighted that the cause of her pain and discomfort had been identified.

Candida albicans presents very real difficulties in stomach and bowel problems. This condition not only depresses the immune system, it also causes allergic reactions and very often this yeast parasite can be the cause of persistent tiredness, lethargy, irritability, abdominal pains, bloatedness and flatulence. Sugar, bread, alcohol, mushrooms or cheese can reactivate a Candida albicans condition, and a persistent craving for any of these foods can be an indication that the condition has been reactivated. Although Candida albicans is dormant in us all, the responsibility of reactiviation is ours. Many women who suffer it also endure bloatedness and flatulence, vaginal burning, thrush or menstrual irregularities. These problems represent only a few of many conditions that can be caused by Candida albicans, which often becomes active after the use of antibiotics – a Candida albicans condition which was thought to have been successfully overcome can recur through using antibiotics for stomach and bowel problems. Simple foods like natural yoghurt, without fruit or colouring, can be of great help. People with Candida tendencies should avoid wine, chocolate, fermented foods, cheese and mushrooms. The elimination of these five items seems to cause many people considerable heartache, and yet they will be handsomely rewarded if they persevere. An active Candida problem nearly always causes allergies. In stomach and bowel problems this yeast parasite floats in the digestive tracts and settles in its favourite sites, the oesophagus and the small intestine, causing harm and affecting the immune system.

Dr Vogel's 'Spring Cleansing Course', which contains four different herbal remedies, is most helpful in cleansing the body thoroughly. I personally take this course twice a year to keep my stomach, bowels, kidneys and liver clear. If you suspect one particular food is causing an allergic reaction, stop eating it for at least three or four weeks, by which time you will know whether you are allergic to this food or not. Recently some interesting tests indicated that food intolerances were often responsible for cases of irritable bowel syndrome.

Food allergies present during infancy can recur with a vengeance at a later stage in life. The best remedy is Harpagophytum, or Devil's Claw, which desensitises the system against all kinds of allergies. Dr Vogel advocates this remedy for the treatment of metabolic dysfunctions, rheumatism and arthritis, liver, gall bladder, kidney and bladder problems and for allergies.

For allergic reactions, especially for stomach and bowel troubles, I may also prescribe Boldocynara, another of Dr Vogel's remedies. This is a fresh herbal preparation for liver and biliary problems, which at the same time stimulates the production of bile. Boldocynara contains:

Cynara scolymus	Artichoke
Carduus marianus	St Mary's thistle
Polygonum aviculare	Knotweed
Taraxacum off.	Dandelion
Peumus boldus	Boldo
Berberis vulgaris	Barberry
Raphanus sativus	Radish
Mentha piperita	Peppermint
Aloe capensis	Aloe
Lycopodium clavatum	Club moss

Finally, whatever the allergy, I nearly always advise the patient to use Nature's Best Imuno-Strength. This is a special formula to help strengthen the immune system, which is distributed throughout the body and is composed of white cells found in the lymph glands, the liver, the spleen, the blood and the bone marrow. There are two main types of white cells, namely granulocytes, which produce an immediate response to a challenge by releasing chemicals, and lymphocytes, which produce a delayed response, adjusting their attack to the new invader, or remembering it from a previous time. There are two types of lymphocytes – B cells which produce antibodies, and T cells which modify this response.

The components of the immune system rely on nutrients in our diet for their production and maintenance. For example, zinc is included because the thymus gland, which produces T cells, relies on this nutrient for its healthy functioning. Included are two herbs, closely associated with the immune system, Echinacea and Harpagophytum. *Echinacea purpurea* is widely cultivated for its gorgeous flowers and has been extensively analysed to identify its active compounds. *Harpagophytum*, or Devil's Claw, is an African plant bearing large, hooked, claw-like fruit. The tuber is widely used for its medicinal properties. A full list of the ingredients in Imuno-Strength is given on page 78.

An important step towards maintaining a healthy immune system is to provide sufficient nutritional support. Imuno-Strength can safeguard the supply of important nutrients when the diet is not all it should be.

In the case of an active Candida albicans condition, Harpagophytum, Imuno-Strength and Molkosan offer the patient the greatest opportunity for recovery. A few months ago I saw a patient who could no longer tolerate her gastrointestinal problems. Tests indicated all the classical symptoms of a Candida problem with a rather ineffective immune system. Together we revised her diet and I prescribed several remedies, and very quickly she improved. She disappointingly remarked that although I had not stipulated very severe dietary restrictions, she was most upset by the 'no chocolate' advice. This was her weakness. However, it did not take her long to notice the benefits to her health condition and she agreed that this was worth far more than the occasional indulgence in some chocolate every now and then. As is so often the case, a simple food item that appears quite innocuous is eventually pinpointed as an offensive substance, and is easily capable of adversely affecting our health.

Chapter 16

Irritable Bowel Syndrome

Now that I have reached the latter stages of this book and I think over the many problems discussed here, somebody of whom I am very fond comes to mind. Never will I forget the despair and anxiety in the eyes of a young woman who had been misdiagnosed and given unsuitable medication for her condition. When I first met her she was almost suicidal. She was a highly intelligent young woman with a responsible position and she was the victim of some dreadful abdominal problems. Only a few of her abdominal organs still functioned: among other problems, her liver, lymphatic, adrenal and bowel functions were severely impaired. She also had a very poor appetite. Her bowels would not move voluntarily and even laxatives were barely effective. Colonic irrigation seemed to be the immediate answer. Even though homoeopathy is a marvellous science, it is of course still dependent upon the knowledge of the practitioner. Ultimately it is his or her decision when and what to prescribe, especially when constitutional remedies are used. One of the reasons that this patient was in such poor condition was that some of the constitutional remedies that had been used had worked against her.

First of all I decided to concentrate on her abdominal problems. She had all the symptoms of an irritable bowel syndrome and, bearing in mind her lack of appetite, the best thing I could prescribe for her was Centaurium. I have already mentioned this remedy for the purpose of stimulating the appetite, and it is also successfully used for anorexia nervosa patients. When this woman's appetite improved, some of the gastric juices started to flow again. As could be expected, the acid and alkaline balance was extremely poor and this is when diet is so very important. A general diet is difficult here, because dietary requirements depend upon individual circumstances. Stress, of course, is an important factor as you will know by now, and mentally she was certainly suffering considerably, because she had no idea what was happening. All she knew for certain was that her health was poor.

As with most of the conditions described in this book, the main contributory factors for irritable bowel syndrome are diet and stress. Scientific research indicates that one out of every six people in the western world will at some time during their life have problems in this respect. The general consensus is that smoking is an aggravating factor in this conditon.

I have already stated that acid is necessary for the digestion process. Acid converts pepsinogen to pepsin, an enzyme that degrades proteins to amino acids, and eventually to glycogen, stored in the liver to maintain the blood-sugar level. It is secreted in response to acetylcholine from the vagus nerve, gastrin from the antrum of the stomach, or from histadine. Each of these substances inhibits its own receptors' parietal cells in the stomach lining. When the two bond together, acid is released, providing the individual's ability to secrete hydrochloric acid is active.

Scientists don't know why, but when something goes wrong too much acid is secreted and it begins to eat into the stomach or duodenum. By 1977 antacids were one of the world's largest selling medical products. It was thought that acid was the culprit, so drugs were developed to inhibit the body's ability to secrete it, but now it is recognised that some acid is necessary to help sterilise bacteria among other things. A gradual decline in the body's production of hydrochloric acid is normal, and by the age of forty most people require a digestive aid. It is recognised that even though antacids may bring relief, they can also cause problems.

In the case of irritable bowel syndrome or spastic colon, which is a disorder involving the small intestine and the large bowel, the symptoms include various degrees of abdominal pain, constipation or diarrhoea. Only too often this is an individual's reaction to stress, and remains a mystery to many physicians. Flatulence, pain and unusually strong intestinal contractions, diarrhoea or constipation may be symptoms of irritable bowel syndrome or a spastic colon. Although I have found it takes considerable effort to reverse this condition, I assure you that it can be overcome.

The young woman mentioned at the start of the chapter had a spastic colon, but because the abdominal organs had been affected a number of remedies were required. Thank goodness for her determination: because of her persistence we managed a considerable improvement, although it will be a long time before she is completely well again. Because of previous mismanagement the organs which have been damaged will take quite a while to mend.

In her excellent book *The Complete Guide to Digestive Health*, Kathleen Mayes writes that smoking is a major contributing factor to irritable bowel syndrome, a conclusion I agree with entirely. Nicotine affects the colon and will definitely have a detrimental influence on a spastic colon. In the case of frequent watery bowel movements immediate medical attention is necessary. A nervous diarrhoea attack, symptomatic of the irritable bowel syndrome, a bout of depression, fatigue or anxiety can trigger off these watery stools. In these cases breathing and relaxation exercises can relieve the stress. Every patient with irritable bowel syndrome will confirm that their symptoms are aggravated during stressful times. I am amazed at the number of people with this problem, and by how often it strikes. Jealousy, divorce, emotional upsets, relationship or financial problems can all cause this problem to flare up quickly. The symptoms are usually similar – flatulence, passing mucus with stools, alternating diarrhoea and constipation, abdominal pain and wind. I have also noticed that bowel and bladder work together in these instances and we see increased frequency of passing water and after a bowel movement the feeling of more to come.

In our clinic we have also noticed that back pain or headaches can be a symptom, or a diminished sex drive, tiredness and anxiety. Many of the problems described in previous chapters contribute to irritable bowel syndrome. One thing is clear: it is certainly not a psychological problem. Too often it is said that it is all in the mind, but irritable bowel syndrome is a real

113

problem that requires sympathetic understanding. The other day I saw a young woman who told me about a sharp, burning abdominal pain, usually experienced after mealtimes. To allay her fears she had come to see me. I explained that when the colon is extended, constipation can occur and her particular symptoms surely showed that she was a victim of irritable bowel syndrome. She told me that her doctor had prescribed anti-spasmodic drugs, which had not changed the situation. I prescribed Nux Vomica which gave her some help, and I also told her about the Hara breathing method which would help her to relax. Hot and cold compresses on the stomach can also work well. Within the first few weeks she reported that these measures had been reasonably successful and that her problems were already diminishing.

The homoeopathic remedies Bryonia or Belladonna are helpful, and another remedy I often prescribe is Ginsavena. This is Dr Vogel's herbal preparation for strengthening and fortifying the nerves. It protects against nervous disorders, lack of concentration and restlessness as well as a general feeling of listlessness. One big mistake this young lady made is that at one stage she had taken large doses of harsh laxatives, and probably as a result, she had also had problems with diarrhoea. The whole bowel was so unbalanced that she did not know what to do anymore. Because avoiding stress is so important, relaxation exercises were helpful and the Hara breathing exercise, which is described in great detail in my book *Stress and Nervous Disorders*, was very useful in this situation.

Osteopathic treatment can also lead to considerable improvement for sufferers of irritable bowel syndrome, as the osteopath may relieve problems in the spine where there is a dysfunction of the disc on the intestines. Bones and muscles harmonise health by means of a system of reflexes and muscle chains, which allows the organs to correctly relax in the abdomen, pelvis and chest cavity. As irritable bowel syndrome is a disorder in which there are abnormal reflexes, an osteopath can balance the automatic nerve pathways in the organs.

Sometimes acupuncture will also help and a well-trained and qualified acupuncturist will know how to ease the problem. Reflexology and aromatherapy treatments can be useful too in these circumstances. The main thing is the belief and the conviction that this problem can be overcome with help and persistence. Too often it is misunderstood and underrated, but it could well be classified as a typical twentieth-century disease.

If constipation appears to be the main symptom of irritable bowel syndrome, I am inclined to prescribe flax-seed oil, a remedy which is currently receiving a great deal of attention from respected nutritionists worldwide. Research has shown it to be the world's richest natural food source of the Omega 3 essential fatty acid alpha-linolenic acid. Flax-seed oil is in fact richer in Omega 3 than fish oils and is therefore an excellent alternative source for these important nutrients that research indicates may be essential for the maintenance of a healthy heart.

Flax (*Linum usitatissimum*) is one of the oldest known cultivated plants, probably originating in the Orient, with small deep-blue flowers and pointed leaves. Flax-seed oil is also known as linseed oil, although this name is normally used to refer to the industrial grade oils. In this form, the oil is usually highly oxidised and thus of little nutritional use.

As an essential nutrient, alpha-linolenic acid is required in relatively large amounts in the diet. A suggested minimum level is 1,500mg a day, compared with other essential nutrients such as calcium, for which the recommended daily intake is 500mg. The optimum intake of alpha-linolenic acid might be as high as 10g per day, depending on the total consumption of fat in the diet. The best sources of the acid are flax-seed (57 per cent), pumpkin seed (15 per cent), unrefined soya oil (9 per cent) and walnut oil (5 per cent), while several vegetables contain small amounts.

Since alpha-linolenic acid is highly unstable and easily destroyed by light, heat and air, it is not always possible to be sure how much is available in the diet. In order to preserve this essential fatty acid, the flax-seed oil from Nature's Best is extracted from organically grown flax and is cold-pressed, without heat and in the absence of light and oxygen, to ensure that the nutritive qualities are retained. The opaque capsules and containers further ensure the extracted oil is protected.

Flax-seed oil is also rich in linoleic acid, which is the 'parent' fatty acid to the Omega fatty acids, for which Evening Primrose is extensively cultivated. Oil of Evening Primrose is a great balancing agent for the body's hormonal functions and for diverse conditions such as breathing problems, fluid retention, fatigue, cystitis and flatulence. With abdominal pains, constipation, anxieties, and mucus in the stools, flax-seed oil is of great help.

I have had several patients with irritable bowel syndrome who have also had problems of hyperventilation. This condition can cause considerable anxiety and in these cases I prescribe Jayvee tablets. This is a most effective remedy, combining Valerian, Crataegus, Humulus, Viscum album, Passiflora, Melissa and zinc. If taken in conjunction with some relaxation exercises, many of the hyperventilation symptoms will soon disappear.

Lastly, I should mention the benefits of peppermint. I have seen very promising results with patients suffering from irritable bowel syndrome. As the majority of sufferers fail to consult their doctor, it is helpful to know that Obbekjaer's Peppermint can be used without fear of any side-effects. I am delighted that nowadays many conventional doctors have realised the value of this preparation. Obbekjaer's Peppermint is available as a tablet or as powder and the results of various tests show that the relief of abdominal pain is indeed very considerable as a result of this remedy. It may not actually be considered a cure, but many people have found that the digestive system improved and pain was relieved. One of my patients, an elderly lady who also had diverticulitis, found that the anti-spasmodic preparation her doctor prescribed did not relieve her discomfort. Yet, this peppermint preparation had the desired effect. The case histories and testimonials I have on this product are quite fascinating.

In the many years I have been in practice I have seen an enormous increase in stomach and bowel disorders. I have come to the conclusion that much of this is induced by the stress caused by our modern lifestyles. Unfortunately, we often conveniently forget that we originate from nature and we should remain true to nature, always remembering that the force of nature is capable of healing us. There are many medical problems that can be overcome naturally and if we decide to follow the natural way, we can rest assured that we need not fear any side-effects. However, professional guidance may be required and sympathetic understanding will be helpful. Dr Vogel quite rightly reminds us that the force of nature will restore equilibirium where mankind has lost the balance. Some of the remedies mentioned, or a change in diet, may be used in a complementary fashion for whatever treatment the patient has been prescribed. Never lose sight of reality and do not despair, because most problems can be overcome; there is no need to suffer unnecessarily. It is so much wiser to seek advice and concentrate on overcoming such conditions, as they may eventually lead to more serious diseases. It is wonderful when the body's chemistry works to such an extent that we can utilise it to the full. It all depends on the type and quality of the nutrients that we feed into it. If these ingredients are wholesome and natural the body will reward us and show us how magnificently generous creation has been.

I admire the perseverance shown by some of my patients. They are prepared to listen and accept advice on dietary management, even though sometimes their diet cannot have been much fun because of the rather severe restrictions that are occasionally necessary. Despite this they remain confident that they will win through in the end. Never forget that no matter how good the treatment, persistence and determination are equally important. The right treatment in the right place is capable of effecting great changes. Be positive and take action and you will reach your goal. In the words of Marcus Aurtius: 'Very little is needed to make a happy and healthy life. It is all within oneself and one's way of thinking.'

Bibliography

Harry Benjamin, *Everybody's Guide to Nature Cure*, Thorsons Publishing Group, Wellingborough

Richard Bircher Benner, *Maag en Darm Klachten*, De Driehoek, Amsterdam, The Netherlands

Paul Bragg, *The Miracle of Fasting*, Health Science, Santa Barbara, USA

Jennifer Britt, *Peppermint*, Silver Link Publishing, Peterborough

Gwynne H. Davies, *Overcoming Allergies*, Ashgrove Press, Bath

Dorothy Hall, *The Natural Health Book*, Nelson Publishing, Melbourne,. Australia

Joan Lay, *Hiatus Hernia*, Thorsons Publishing Group, Wellingborough

Kathleen Mayes, *The Complete Guide to Digestive Health*, Thorsons Publishing Group, Wellingborough

Leonard Mervyn, *Stomach Ulcers and Acidity*, Thorsons Publishing Group, Wellingborough

Rosemary Nicol, *Coping Successfully with Irritable Bowel Syndrome*, Sheldon Press, London

Shirley Tricket, *Irritable Bowel Syndrome*, HarperCollins, London

Alfred Vogel, *The Nature Doctor*, Mainstream, Edinburgh

Arthur White, *Colitis*, Thorsons Publishing Group, Wellingborough

Arthur White, *Diverticulitis*, Thorsons Publishing Group, Wellingborough

Useful Addresses

Bioforce (UK) Ltd, Olympic Business Park, Dundonald, KA2 9BE
Nature's Best, Freepost PO Box 1, Tunbridge Wells, TN2 3EQ
Auchenkyle, Southwoods Road, Troon, Ayrshire, KA19 7EL
Obbekjaers, 209 Blackburn Road, Wheelton, Chorley, Lancs

Index